INFERTILITY
SUCCESS

Stories of Help and Hope
for Your Journey

By

Erica Hoke

Introduction by Martha Huie

Constance Lewis, Diane Prunier, Susan Tozer,
Brandi Bunda, Cindy Grace, Kaila Stearns,
Laura Watson, Saskia Williams, Amanda Ignot,
Cindy D. Vochatzer-Murillo, Amber Stier,
Jacci Robyn Lötter, Drew Jacobs, Jules Batchelor,
Kendra Becker, Nancy Powell, Jaida Schupp,
Jennifer Tunny

CONTENTS

INTRODUCTION

Martha Huie, AP

In these chapters you will see many of the women utilized acupuncture and traditional Chinese medicine (TCM) in their journey to conceive. Patients come for acupuncture because a friend, family member, or colleague tells them to try it. Early in my career, I often said I practice in the "theatre of last resort," since other medical modalities had not been successful. Now, acupuncture and herbs are part of the "mainstream" of options for many medical issues, including infertility.

When I endured menopause 30 years ago, no effective solutions were forthcoming for the flashes, the general malaise, and the intense irritability! In desperation, I went for acupuncture. Astonished and relieved, I felt the symptoms of menopause fade away. I kept regular acupuncture appointments and kept asking questions because I felt so much better. Finally, the acupuncture physician said, "I have enrolled you in school!"

As a result of my own experience, I planned to focus my acupuncture practice on mid-life issues for women, but that did not happen. I was treating tennis elbows, frozen shoulders, headaches, migraines, colds/flu, and **infertility**.

Traditional Chinese medicine (TCM) has a vast and venerable history of treating the entire person: body, mind, and spirit, not just symptoms of illness. For millennia, the Chinese physicians kept detailed medical records and data. I studied both here in the U.S. and in China. My professors were both western doctors and TCM doctors. I have a wealth of knowledge upon which to draw to help my patients.

Traditional Chinese medicine diagnoses and treats the cause of a condition, not just the symptom. There are many factors that can cause infertility: poor diet, irregular menses, excessive exercise routines, extreme work hours, stress, age, POCS, genetics, anemia, and general health, to name a few.

One happy story I can relate after acupuncture treatments for a patient: Erica Hoke and I were walking to an outdoor function of the Sarasota Chamber of Commerce. I took her hand as we were walking across the grass. One of her pulses was very strong, and I said, "You are pregnant! ... and it's a boy!" She said the stick test had not registered yet. "Does not matter, the pulse knows." Nine months later, her son was born.

Pregnancy is a special time for women to focus on self-care. Adjust lifestyle choices and habits to prevent a miscarriage. Avoid stress as much as possible! Allow and plan time for additional personal pleasures: afternoon naps, favorite snacks, relaxing dinners, happy movies, and only gentle walks!

TCM is regulatory in nature and brings the body, mind and spirit back into balance. Over the years, I have tried to assist patients in managing lifestyle decisions and habits to facilitate conception, in addition to acupuncture and herbs. This medicine is unique in that it treats each patient individually; one size does not fit all. Some pregnancies are the result of the combination of both Asian and western medicines (IVF and IUI). The length of treatment varies as well. One of our patients conceived after one acupuncture session, but for others, 4-6 months might be needed.

TCM offers so much more than just assistance in conception protocols. Menstrual issues, morning sickness, assistance with delivery, insomnia, anxiety, and postpartum depression are successfully treated. Fathers may also need help with sperm count, motility, and morphology, and TCM is helpful in these areas.

I want to express my deepest gratitude to Dr. Hui Luo, who is an OBGYN, an acupuncture physician with a PhD in fertility. She generously shared her knowledge and expertise with me. She taught me about many other aspects and benefits of TCM as well as fertility.

We are thrilled for our mothers as they conceive their babies (three sets of twins in our clinic!). We attend the baby showers, bring diapers, and provide some guidance with delivery. As I looked over our book with the baby pictures, one young mother wrote, "Thank you so much for all you have done to help bring this miracle to life." Our care is personal, and I am honored to be the godmother of one of the twins.

I was taught that it is a privilege to practice traditional Chinese medicine, and I am grateful we could offer the many special benefits of TCM to our fertility patients.

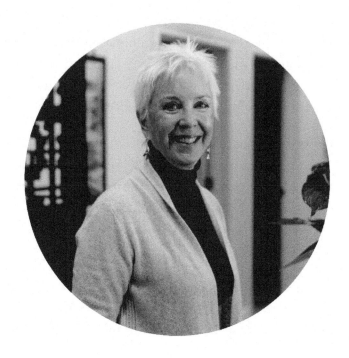

Martha Huie, AP, has a passion for helping people and spreading knowledge about Traditional Chinese Medicine.

Martha Huie, AP, is the founder and owner of Acupuncture Anywhere and is licensed as an acupuncture physician by the state of Florida.

Initially, she pursued a traditional western education including a bachelor of arts degree from the College of William and Mary and a masters in fine arts at Virginia Commonwealth University. She fulfilled her academic and clinical requirements at the East West College of Natural Medicine in Sarasota, Florida. Martha has also studied traditional Chinese medicine in China at Zhejiang University.

Professionally trained in theatre, Martha is an engaging speaker on radio, television and before live audiences. Her knowledge of traditional Chinese medicine is extensive and she makes the topic accessible to all audiences.

http://acupunctureanywhere.net

SEVEN DIAGNOSES AND SEVEN YEARS TO FOUR SONS

Erica Hoke

f ever there was a woman that was least likely to conceive, it was me. I was over age 35 when I was diagnosed with stage four endometriosis, uterine fibroids, PCOS, thyroid disease, low ferritin, low ovarian reserve, and factor 5 leiden. With seven contributing infertility diagnoses, I was still considered to have "unexplained infertility." In the back of my mind, IVF was a choice of last resort, or at least it was a choice... until it wasn't.

My husband and I sat in the reproductive endocrinologist office. "You're 35, and you're already hyper-ovulating. Your body is already doing the job that medicine we give you would do. The ultrasound and bloodwork show you have very few eggs left."

"I'm sorry," he said. "You have a better chance of hitting the lottery than getting pregnant." The only option the REI could offer us was IUI, which carried a less than five percent chance of success. Those odds weren't good enough for us, especially since, at that point, we knew my husband's swimmers were "Olympic" level. That's when I started researching anything and everything that affects fertility and then implementing these changes.

TIP: If you're given a poor prognosis with few choices, get another opinion.

That "no" to IVF treatment from our REI wasn't the beginning of our journey. We had been traveling a path to find answers and heal my body from my many reproductive diagnoses for several years. But to understand the full picture, you have to know that my problems started a few years after my first period.

The first memory of the intensity of my periods increasing was Thanksgiving. I rushed from the table to throw up and spent the day in bed. At sixteen, just three years after starting my period, this was "normal" for the first day of my cycle.

The gynecologist offered a prescription for an NSAID and the platitude that the pain was "normal."

TIP: Extreme period pain that includes vomiting, an inability to stand upright, or causes you to miss school or work is not normal and requires additional investigation to determine the medical root cause.

Years later, I was able to see the pattern of what I believed caused the disease that took doctors 15 years to diagnose.

I met my husband one day on a sales call for my job. We were both divorced with no children. When we met, we were both in our early to mid-30s. As our relationship progressed and we spent more time together, he was able to see first-hand what I dealt with on a monthly basis.

Over the 15+ years of having my period, I dealt with the pain mostly by being on hormonal birth control. Convinced this was causing a lot of other symptoms, I decided to stop using it. I was concerned about the long-term effects on my fertility and determined to get my body in the best possible health to carry a baby.

Within months of stopping the pill, my pain had increased to an excruciating level. I was working in outside sales, and my flow was nearly impossible to manage. During a networking lunch, I met a traditional Chinese medicine doctor who practiced acupuncture and would change the course of my life. She assured me that she could help me. It seemed like as soon as I found help, my body went on attack. More than once, my then-boyfriend had to deliver me to her office for treatment while I was sobbing and unable to stand.

In addition to acupuncture, my new gynecologist, although amazing, was ethically bound to only be able to tell me my symptoms *could be* endometriosis or uterine fibroids. Diagnosis meant surgery. Eventually, unable to get relief, I sought out a surgeon who specializes in endometriosis. I was terrified the surgery would cause scarring in my uterus that would prevent me from getting pregnant.

*TIP: If your doctor suspects endometriosis or uterine fibroids, **don't delay** confirming the diagnosis with surgery. DO find a surgeon that will diagnose AND perform the surgical excision at the same surgery.*

We discussed what would happen if she found endometriosis. She let me know that she was one of the few surgeons who would perform the laparoscopic surgery *and* perform the excision surgery. After lots of talking it over and consideration, I decided to have the surgery.

When I woke up from the surgery, the surgeon said she removed *a lot* of endometrioses, stage 4 endometriosis, to be exact. It was the diagnosis I had been waiting 15 years for. It was both inside and outside of my uterus, attached to my ovaries, bladder, and bowels. She was able to see I also had PCOS.

She felt confident that, because of her aggressive surgery, most, if not all, of my problems would be over. She was wrong. While grateful for her skill as a surgeon, the next few months would be some of the most trying of my journey up until that point.

> *TIP: Before any surgical procedure, any doctor should complete a basic blood panel to confirm your overall health.*

Bleeding was to be expected for a few weeks following the surgery, but when a month went by, and my bleeding hadn't stopped, I contacted the surgeon. She sent me home with no suggestions and a "wait and see" attitude. The pain was gone, but for the next 90+ days, I had period-like flow. Little did I know, I was literally bleeding to death.

> *TIP: If any doctor tells you they can't help you with a problem that seems concerning to you or is disruptive to your life, get a second opinion or keep doing your own research until you find an answer.*

I was back to work full time, but I was exhausted. I went to work and came home and headed straight for the couch. Around this time, I drove out of town for work. When I got to the event, I had so much pain in my leg that I couldn't walk. Something was wrong.

A few days later, a red, belt strap looking welt appeared on my leg. I went to see my doctor. After some discussion and hesitation, he decided to send me to the hospital for the ultrasound I didn't receive days earlier when I visited the ER. The ultrasound was inconclusive, and I was admitted to the hospital.

I was so afraid and freaked out. At 33, I was being admitted to the hospital for the first time. The doctor ordered blood work and blood thinners "just in case" I had a blood clot in my leg. A nurse came in to get my blood thinners started, and I was making small talk with her when a tiny voice in my head sounded an alarm.

TIP: If you have an intuition about something or feel something is off, trust your instinct. Always confirm and ask to see any medication being given to you in the hospital.

I looked over at the tray **full** of small vials she was steadily pushing into my IV. I asked, *"Are you going to give me all of that?"* It was a question that saved my life. She looked at me and told me that she would be right back. I never saw her again during my 10-day hospital stay. Instead, a male nurse bustled into the room with an IV pole with a bag of vitamin K hung on it, the antidote to blood thinners.

I had been overdosed by a whole decimal point. Had I not noticed, my organs and brain would have liquefied before the antidote could have been administered.

The lab results revealed that I had a gene mutation called factor 5 leiden. According to a local geneticist, up to 80% of the population is a carrier. If not diagnosed, it leads to chemical pregnancy, miscarriage, still birth, and secondary infertility. Ultimately, this diagnosis would allow me to go on to hold and carry my pregnancies. Along with this diagnosis came hope.

Tip: If you have had even one miscarriage, or suspect chemical pregnancies, get tested for a blood clotting panel, especially factor 5 leiden.

In addition, I also had an undiagnosed thyroid issue causing my continuous bleeding from the surgery. Because of my blood loss, my red blood count was 2 points away from being fatal.

Diagnosed and back on the road to health with my now-fiancé, I knew that I still had some problems to solve. The endometriosis surgery had eliminated most (but not all) of my pain but not the torrential flow that became the norm. I sought out our town's only reproductive endocrinologist that specializes in infertility to get recommendations on next steps. He recommended my gynecologist perform a laparoscopic surgery to determine/remove any fibroids he could see.

The laparoscopic surgery was unsuccessful. My OB/GYN couldn't see a single fibroid to remove. Seeing my anguish, he let me know that there might be another type of fibroid surgery that could be done by the REI to be certain that I didn't have any fibroids. He explained that when looking into the uterus, the fibroids might be receding into the wall of the uterus. A saline infusion sonogram would allow the surgeon to see the fibroids better.

Bounced back to my REI, I scheduled the surgery as soon as I could. I was willing to do whatever it took to get to the bottom of my pain. When I woke up, I was shocked by the news the surgeon had for me.

Not only did he find that I DID, in fact, have fibroids, he removed so many that it looked like a handful of aquarium gravel. I was horrified because all that I could think about was whether or not each fibroid scar would be one less piece of real estate in my uterus but also thrilled because I was hopeful that this meant I would be pain-free.

Now, with the endo and fibroids gone, I *was sure* we were on a short path to parenthood. One month went by and then two. I was pain-free and having normal cycles now but more concerned than ever about the ticking clock and no pregnancy.

Now that my problems were cleared up, I started to question if something could be wrong with my husband. No one ever suggested my husband be tested for male factor infertility.

TIP: Request as much testing up front as you can. Even if you have to pay out of pocket for it. Don't wait (for time, miscarriages, or failed IVF/IUI) to start procedures/testing. Don't wait to test your partner until issues with you are ruled out.

My husband got a glowing report on his swimmers, and we were back to the drawing board.

During our next two week wait, we decided to splurge and take a combined birthday/anniversary trip to Disney to relax and take a break from all thing's fertility-related (at least the painful ones). We ate a lot of good food, drank a lot of good wine, and then, at Epcot, got on the world's largest centrifuge (in the form of the ride Mission Space).

When we returned home, I went straight to acupuncture treatment. Afterward, Dr. H. and I decided to attend a chamber of commerce function. As we were walking around the different tables, she reached over to grab my hand and feel my pulse. She stopped dead in her tracks and turned to face me squarely, still gripping my wrist. "You're pregnant! and it's a boy!"

"What?!" I say, "I haven't even taken a pregnancy test." It was several more days of waiting before I was brave enough to confirm the prediction. We WERE pregnant and over the moon with excitement! It was my first positive pregnancy test ever.

Once the pregnancy was confirmed and the blood thinners on board to prevent a clot, we went about our business in the manner of any new and excited parents. I continued to work and, although monitored very closely, didn't have any scares, minus some spotting during an out-of-town business trip. It was a perfectly uneventful pregnancy.

We welcomed our first son after a 28-hour labor prevented him from being born on Christmas Day. I was 36.

After 15 months with a *super easy* baby, we were convinced that we were genius parents and ready to expand our family. We knew from the start that we wanted as many children as the Lord would allow us to have.

We returned to the same REI (in hindsight, I'm not sure why), and he had an even bleaker prognosis for us. After two and a half years, my blood work, including my AMH, was terrible. When he looked at my follicle count via ultrasound, he declared that I would need donor eggs in order to conceive. I think we were both stunned with disbelief.

My husband and I never even talked about using donor eggs as an option. Instead, we decided to drive an hour away for a second opinion. Unfortunately, this doctor wasn't any more optimistic about my outcome. He *did*, however, suggest that I take the blood thinners that I would need during pregnancy before we got a positive pregnancy test. He handed me a prescription and sent us on our way. It was Tuesday, and we were in our two week wait window.

Friday, I woke up feeling optimistic enough to take an early test. Much to my surprise, it was positive!!!! I couldn't believe my eyes. I rushed to the pharmacy to fill my prescription and schedule an ultrasound with my doctor.

While I was caring for our not quite two-year-old and waiting for the ultrasound, my husband noticed that I often referred to the pregnancy as "they" or "them." Hmm. That's weird, I thought. I wonder why I'm doing that? Both my husband and I had prophetic dreams about having twin girls.

Finally, it was ultrasound day, and we relayed our suspicions to the doctor. "Nope, just one baby here." We weren't disappointed and just blew it off. We were happily pregnant again.

I was very sick very early in the pregnancy. I had an ultrasound scheduled, but my husband stayed home (the only ultrasound he ever missed) with our son, who had the sniffles. The doctor placed the ultrasound wand on my stomach, and as the screen lit up, there were two "fried egg" images on the screen. It was the top of both my sons' heads. "That looks like twins!" I said. "It sure does!" he replied. Our prediction was correct.

Our twin boys were born at 39 weeks, 27 months after the birth of their big brother, one vaginally and one via c-section. I wouldn't change a thing about the outcome of our birth experience. Happy as a family of five, we struggled through our first year of twin life and then hit our stride the second year.

One morning, one of the boys woke me up. We had just returned from vacation, and my husband was gone on a business trip. The night before, I'd realized that I lost track of my period, and I reminded myself that when one of the boys woke in the morning, I would take a pregnancy test I had left over, "just in case." I peed on the stick, set it aside, and went to care for my son, almost forgetting on my way back to bed that I hadn't looked at it.

I was unconcerned, after all of our previous tracking, that this could be a "surprise" pregnancy. After all, I was 41. I flipped on the light and was STUNNED to see two dark lines staring back at me. We were pregnant! WOW. The birth would be the exact same spacing as the first two. Twenty-seven months.

The pregnancy was problematic from the start. First of all, it was the Friday before Labor Day weekend. I phoned the office as soon as they opened to make sure I got my blood thinner medicine before the weekend. It didn't happen. They closed at noon. It would be late the following week before they could see me.

Despite my panic, I tried to tell myself that it would be okay. I was wrong. By the time I was seen for my first appointment, they couldn't detect a heartbeat. They sent me to the hospital for a second detailed ultrasound, and I learned that I miscarried not one but two babies. We will always feel like that was our twin girls.

The miscarriage was devastating. Busy with the boys and convinced that another pregnancy was out of the question, we gave accidental pregnancy very little thought. Now, we were determined this miscarriage would not be how our story ended.

Months passed and then the year anniversary of the miscarriage. I was 42 and needed surgery to correct a severe diastasis rectus from the twin's pregnancy (combined, I carried over 12 pounds of baby) that left me looking five months pregnant on my size 4 frame.

We set a deadline of January 1st, 2015, to stop trying. I would be 43 that year and needed closure. I had given up hope. Seventeen months after the loss of our twins, and just two days before our "deadline," we got our positive pregnancy test!

After another uneventful pregnancy, I delivered, via unmedicated VBAC, our last son. It was truly a redemptive experience. We call him our 11th hour baby.

We welcomed our fourth son **SEVEN** years after medical professionals told us that we would not be able to conceive on our own or would need donor eggs. There are a lot of procedures/surgeries and details I was not able to include here due to space constraints. Some of these include massive changes in my diet, including switching to organic proteins, then organic veggies, then low/no processed foods. I eliminated soda from my diet, which is a killer to gut health (gut health is foundational to your hormones). I had a hysterosalpingography (HSG), which I believe helped "unblock" my tubes by proxy. There were two iron IV infusion treatments due to low ferritin (but normal iron levels). I outline all the steps that I believe helped me conceive and all that I've learned since then, in my course by the same name -- "Infertility Success." I'm determined to help as many women as I can get to the families of their dreams.

Also not mentioned, the emotional toll month after month of grieving as my period appeared and reappeared. Not to mention months of faking a smile and shrugging off intrusive questions to get through my job. When our oldest son was one, I went on hiatus from my very stressful sales job and, two months later, conceived our twins. It was a financial sacrifice that took us years of adjustments to recover from, but I 100% believe it contributed to their conception.

Only after the fact, and years later, did I realize that I had many, many chemical pregnancies. There were always the tell-tale signs and symptoms of pregnancy, and then I would get my cycle, and they faded away.

> *TIP: Don't discount the little things (coffee, toxins, dehydration, gut health, sleep, stress, exercise); all can dramatically affect the outcome of your procedure and getting pregnant on your own.*

I'll leave you with this. If a doctor tells you **they** can't help you, it doesn't mean you can't get pregnant. I didn't get pregnant because I was special, but because I was willing to exhaust any and all obstacles to build the family of our dreams.

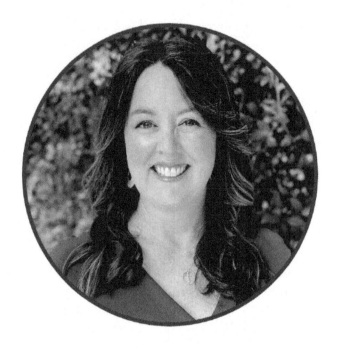

Scan the code for a video message from Erica and a free gift

Erica Hoke is the infertile mother of 4 boys, all born to her as a "geriatric" pregnant lady. After struggling for years with undiagnosed endometriosis, uterine fibroids, PCOS, thyroid disease, factor 5 Leiden and low ovarian reserve, unable to participate in traditional IUI or IVF methods, she was able to get to the bottom of her infertility issues via continual changes to her diet and lifestyle.

Now she fiercely shares her story and the stories of others as a means to give hope to those still on the path to creating the family of their dreams. Dissatisfied with the way reproductive endocrinology

(REI) medicine handles common infertility issues, Erica is determined to disrupt the entire reproductive medical system. Empowering infertility patients by creating a standard of care and testing path through which to collaborate and coordinate with their doctors has become her mission. This approach allows the patients to systematically address and remove all obstacles before pursuing invasive and expensive IUI and IVF treatments.

Erica mentors' clients through the infertility process via a free support group, group coaching, courses to address diet, toxins and lifestyle that affect infertility, and one on one coaching.

STRUCK BY LIGHTNING

Constance Lewis, BSN, MSN, WHNP

There is a constant balancing act between luck and choices while struggling with infertility. I had more than my fair share of "bad luck." As my doctor said, "lightning struck us multiple times." Blaming myself early on, as many women do, limited me from seeing other causes and choosing alternative options. There were moments throughout my 8-year-long journey when I considered giving up.

The infertility process was suffocating and isolating. I found it hard to allow anyone else to help lighten the load of emotional, physical, and spiritual pain. I thought that no one else could understand or relate. It's the woman's job to get pregnant and carry the baby. So, therefore, my job was to carry the burden.

Since the focus was on me, *that is what cost us the most money and why it took longer to become pregnant.* The woman's body is also the focus for a fertility provider. It would have been beneficial if our provider would have seen us as a whole unit, testing us both.

> *TIP: Insist that your provider look at the couple as a whole for testing and possible reasons for infertility.*

At 29 years old, and being "type A," I expected to be pregnant right away. Two weeks later, when my period started, I was surprised and sad. We decided to give it six months before worrying. In my heart, I knew it was the logical thing; however, I already felt something was wrong.

> *TIP: Always trust your instinct.*

My basic infertility testing and knowledge was minimal at first. I used ovulation testing in the first year and never got a positive ovulation test. At no point did my provider ask me if I was getting positive ovulation tests. My OBGYN ordered fertility labs, a hysterosalpingogram (HSG), and a semen sample from my husband.

I was in school to become a women's health nurse practitioner. I had fertility labs drawn, and my nurse practitioner told me all my labs were normal. They were not! I had trusted my nurse practitioner. It's important for patients to see their own lab results, understand what they mean, and know if they are abnormal. If I had not done this, I would have missed a crucial problem.

> *TIP: It's important to see all your diagnostic testing results and know what is normal and what is not.*

My labs were ***not normal***, my anti-müllerian hormone (AMH) level was 0.13, significantly low, devastatingly low. I just sat there, staring at the number in disbelief and having a mini panic attack!

We decided to have ALL of the diagnostic testing. My husband's semen sample was normal. Because his sample was normal -- normal amount, mobility, and motility -- no further testing was requested. No blood chromosome test was done on either of us.

I had an unsuccessful HSG due to the inability of the radiologist or my doctor to pass the catheter to push the dye. After a long conversation about my 9-year history of pelvic pain, a laparoscopy and hysteroscopy were scheduled. I was misdiagnosed multiple times -- heavy cycles, irritable bowel syndrome, interstitial cystitis, and ovarian cysts. I was once told the pain was in my head. The laparoscopy revealed stage I and II endometriosis, and my left ovary was attached to my bladder. It was hard for me to believe that something was wrong after all. Endometriosis was causing my pain. *I wasn't crazy.*

Now, I was diagnosed with both low AMH level and endometriosis. The doctor said the chances of getting pregnant might be improved after the removal of the endometriosis, but based on my level, he recommended intrauterine insemination (IUI). I went on Clomid, a medication to help me ovulate, and started my IUIs. We completed two IUIs in my doctor's office; neither was successful, and I was referred to a fertility specialist.

The ultrasound confirmed that my low AMH level was accurate. I only had six follicles total. We had another IUI using Clomid and a medicated trigger shot. *I wondered if it was wasting my money due to having such a low follicle count;* however, I had seen others in my practice getting pregnant with a low AMH and low follicle count. We continued on with the recommendation.

I remember feeling somewhat hopeful each time going in for the IUI, but then, my period would start. I can't remember why we decided to do so many IUIs before discussing in-vitro fertilization (IVF). Maybe we just weren't mentally ready or we were being pushed by the reproductive endocrinologist (REI). Each IUI cost $500. Six IUIs and a lot of lost hope later, we were ready to move to IVF. After meeting with the financial counselor and swallowing the thought of paying $30,000, the payment for IVF was made.

With our first IVF stimulation, we had six follicles growing. I had gotten used to giving myself injections and was looking forward to the actual egg retrieval. My belly was bruised from all the shots. I was on an emotional roller-coaster, and the hormones made it worse. I just kept telling myself, "You can do this - keep going - it's for a good cause." When I woke up, my first words were, "How many eggs did they get?" We got six eggs! It was a good number for my low AMH level. We went back to the hospital with excitement for a day five fresh embryo transfer (a recommendation by my doctor). Two embryos were transferred, and I was sent home to relax.

After the first hCG draw, I got the call that I was pregnant. I was in disbelief; I couldn't believe it actually worked! My second HCG was rising! My six-week ultrasound was scheduled. I didn't really feel pregnant. This made me worried, but I knew not all women have symptoms.

I was excited the day we drove to the fertility clinic for the six weeks ultrasound. We got our phone out to record the first ultrasound. The doctor was looking all around, and because of my training, I could read the ultrasound. In disbelief, I knew immediately something was wrong. I told my husband to stop filming.

The doctor told me that things didn't look normal. He said there should be a fetal heartbeat, and the fetus should look bigger. I felt like somebody stabbed me in the heart with a knife. I couldn't breathe; I sobbed the entire way home. I didn't move from the couch for three days, not wanting to talk to anyone. It was gut wrenching. My husband held me. I knew he was taking it hard as well, but he was so strong for me. He said that he felt helpless in that moment.

A few weeks later, I had a conversation with my girlfriend. Tears streaming down my face, I said, "My husband should just leave me. He could have a baby with someone else."

Her eyes watered, and she hugged me. "No!" she shouted! "That's not true; he loves you so much, and you both will do this together."

The emotional pain made me think my husband would have been better off with someone else. That's how isolated I felt.

Around 8 weeks, I realized that the baby wasn't getting bigger, and there was no heartbeat. It was a nightmare that had come true. I wasn't going to pass the fetus on my own, so I let my doctor know that I wanted to have a dilation and curettage (D&C) to remove the baby.

A two-month recovery led to a second transfer with two embryos that had made it to day 6. At this point, we still had not done any genetic testing of the embryos. I tried my best to not get my hopes up. I told myself I was being realistic. No other labs or recommendations had been made for further testing after the first miscarriage.

After the second transfer, my first blood test came back with an hCG of 130. Two days later, it came back 1000. Again, I was excited but also skeptical. Two weeks later, at about 5 1/2 weeks, we did an ultrasound. No intrauterine pregnancy was seen, and then, there was **a negative** repeat hCG and more devastation.

TIP: Again, listen to your instincts.

We decided to try one more IVF retrieval. My follicles were not responding well. In my head, I knew I should have cancelled the retrieval; however, I just couldn't stop. I think I learned, after this, to listen to my gut feeling, no matter what the doctor encouraged. I had ignored so many feelings prior to this, and I was doing it again.

The doctor said to me, "We can do the retrieval, but it's not looking good; I'll leave it up to you." *I wish* he would have just said, "This is not going to work, so let's try again with another cycle." I had already taken the medications and spent the time and energy, so I continued. I got two embryos. My husband said, as he cupped my face, "We only need one."

This time, the doctor said he would freeze the embryos and do genetic testing since I had two miscarriages previously. I didn't hear from anybody on day five, and I finally called the office on day six. The doctor apologized, saying that both embryos had perished, and someone should have notified me sooner.

At this point, I was furious. I couldn't believe that, "Oh, somebody had just forgotten to call and tell me." These are my eggs, *my last two*; these were my future babies, and they didn't even have the decency to call and tell me! My last hope of using my eggs was a forgotten call. The anger filled my soul for months. I felt like just a number, just another large payment to a fertility clinic. All I could think was, "It's done; I'm never having children." I've wasted all this money and time, went through all these miscarriages and pain for nothing.

TIP: Genetically test all of your embryos.

The doctor suggested chromosome testing, *a simple blood test.* I've gone through **six IUIs, two IVF,** and subsequent miscarriages, and NOW recommending a blood test? I thought this should have been suggested with our *initial labs.*

My husband's results were abnormal. He had a chromosome condition called *balance translocation.* I was shocked to hear that my

25

husband had something wrong. I couldn't help but think that if we had known this all along, we could have saved so much heartbreak and money. We would have completed genetic testing on all the embryos before implanting them. That would have saved me two miscarriages! A whole year of my life and multiple nights of crying myself to sleep hinged on "a" simple blood test.

My husband and I had a long discussion that night, his eyes filled with tears, and he said, "See? There is something wrong with me, and I can finally carry the burden of infertility with you." That made me so sad; I didn't want anyone else to feel the burden that I felt. It should have given me some relief, but it didn't. He was overlooked during the infertility testing.

After so many disappointments, we had a great deal of mistrust with our fertility clinic. We decided to find a different clinic. By this time, I had lost so much hope, and I could barely muster the energy to give them a call to make the free appointment.

At the new clinic, the doctors took our case due to the complexity. I remember when I talked to the physician, he said to me, "Wow, you both have been struck by lightning twice, with your low AMH and endometriosis and his balance translocation." Based on all that, he recommended we look into their egg donor program.

I noticed a major difference in the organization, communication, and way we were welcomed into the practice, compared to our original fertility clinic. It felt like a well-oiled machine (in a good way), one that made us feel like part of the family. The doctor that we had been assigned was compassionate and informative. He was available to answer all our questions, and we never felt rushed. I instantly felt more comfortable and understood.

They require anyone that does the donor program to have a therapy session. I thought it was one of the most caring and thoughtful requirements. They were very concerned about our mental health and overall decision about using a donor egg.

I was so torn that I would have to use a donor egg and that I would never ever have a child that had my genetics. In the back of my head, I was thinking that my husband, the man that I fell in love with, and I would never have a baby mixed with our genes. The most impactful thing the counselor at the fertility clinic told me was, "You will be this baby's biological mother." She continued, "You may not be the genetic mother, but this baby cannot live or breathe without your body, without your soul. You will be a biological mother." That was a tremendous, eye-opening statement, and that alone helped me come to grips and cope with the fact that I'd be using a donor egg. Those statements gave me the will to continue my fertility journey.

The clinic recommended a donor that had done an egg retrieval before, one we knew had a good history of numerous eggs on retrieval. I spent three weeks looking at the donor database, thinking I would find the perfect match (the one that looked just like me). I realized that this wasn't going to happen early on. I really had wanted to find someone that WAS me. My heart ached the first few months we searched for a donor.

Eventually, I settled on a girl that had never been a donor before, but I felt a connection with her picture. I remember getting the call from our nurse the day of her retrieval, stating that, unfortunately, the donor only got six embryos and all were abnormal.

I remember going back to the website multiple times a day, seeing if they had added anyone else. We found someone, finally, and she went through the IVF process and got 16 eggs. That eventually dwindled down to six embryos that were viable. We had them frozen and sent off for genetic and chromosome testing.

After the difficult two week wait, a call confirmed ONE good embryo. We were relieved but also nervous because we thought, "What happens if this one egg doesn't work, if we put the embryo in and I have a miscarriage?" We were grateful but also cautious at the same time. My husband looked at me again and said, "It just takes one, babe."

The result was a positive pregnancy test and cautious hope and two normal hCGs. Nervous but more hopeful than ever, the ultrasound revealed a fetal pole and a heartbeat. There was an actual fetus with a heartbeat. Tears filled my eyes, and I sighed in relief.

I had some spotting early on, and I remember sobbing hysterically, thinking that I was having another miscarriage. Luckily, the pregnancy progressed. It didn't feel real, and I found it hard to find a connection to the baby, which made me feel guilty. I was able to convince myself I was happy. I wish someone would have told me that the constant fear of losing the baby and not connecting to the baby was normal after all the losses I had been through. I wish someone would have helped me grieve more -- the loss of my eggs, the loss of my ability to be a genetic mother.

TIP: Find ways to grieve your losses; it will help your future pregnancies and postpartum journeys.

Miracle Miles came into this world mid-December. We call him Miracle Miles because he was the only embryo we got, and against all odds, he came into this world healthy. I finally had a baby I could hold, smell, and kiss.

We knew we wanted another baby but had zero embryos left. Our previous donor was no longer available. This devastated me more than I thought it would. I wanted them to be genetically the same. For two months, I contemplated not even trying for another baby because of this. I felt sad, mad, and frustrated. After a lot of counseling and a lot of talks with my husband, we decided that we did truly want another baby.

TIP: Once you become pregnant, to ensure a full blood sibling, consider freezing embryos with the same donor.

The donor we chose had a fantastic response to IVF, and we got nine healthy embryos, another successful transfer, and a healthy fetus with a heartbeat! Once again, at five weeks, I had bright red bleeding. I remember sitting on the side of the tub and crying. My son looked up at me and said, "Mama, it's okay," while wiping the tears from my eyes.

To my relief, the baby looked good on the ultrasound. They concluded that the embryo had split, and I was to have twins, but the one twin miscarried. After a full-term pregnancy, Mariah arrived, a girl! I had another baby of my own to hold, smell, and kiss.

Although there were many hurdles and things that could've been changed for the better, I have the children I have because of those hurdles. I would've saved a lot of money and heartbreak if I had read this book. I was robbed of the chance to use my own embryos. When I think about that, it makes me sad and, at times, mad. But I also feel this journey brought me *my* two children. I was meant to be *their* mother. I have learned so much and now can help, support, and educate others. It has formed me into the nurse practitioner that I am. I can be there for others in their infertility struggles.

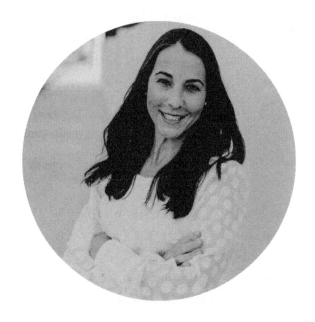

Scan the code for a video message from Constance and a free gift

Constance Lewis is the ultimate worker, grinding her way through degrees and careers as she found her way to her true passion: women's healthcare, gynecology and obstetrics. Beginning that journey as a neonatal ICU nurse in 2004 sparked her pursuit for over a decade. Lewis served as a neonatal nurse, educator, manager, childbirth educator, breastfeeding counselor and then ultimately, graduated with a master of science in nursing education and has since been a practicing nurse practitioner at an OB/GYN practice since 2015. This journey uniquely coincided with her own personal infertility struggle, a struggle that might have been insurmountable except for the determination that served her well in her career. Her passion for supporting women through her work as a NP, specifically women who struggle with infertility, has never subsided, even after she and her husband have been blessed with two children. Outside of her family and career, she enjoys CrossFit, traveling, and spending time with family and friends.

https://womenandbabies.net/

A JOURNEY OF HOPE: SECONDARY INFERTILITY

Diane Prunier

'll never forget that moment. It was a chilly day in mid-December of 2016. The ultrasound technician looked at me with sadness in her eyes and confirmed, "I'm so sorry. There is no heartbeat. I will be right back with the doctor."

I let out a true guttural "Nooooooo!" as I started to cry and held onto my husband, Josh's, hand, staring at the twelve-week outline of our baby on the screen. We were in shock and disbelief as a miscarriage was not something we had ever worried about. It was then that we lost our innocence about how easy it was to have a baby.

Adam, my one-year-old son, had gone with us that day and was squirming in his chair next to Josh. Josh hugged him to help ease the tension which calmed him down. I couldn't believe I was living this moment. It was just supposed to be a routine twelve-week check-up. Instead, when they couldn't find the heartbeat on the doppler, we had an ultrasound to double check if our baby was still alive.

The doctor reassured us that it was not our fault. The baby had passed sometime between eleven and twelve weeks. Since I was that far along, the doctor suggested that I have a D&C (dilation and curettage) the following day. We decided we would do the surgical procedure, and after the doctor gave us some information, he left us alone in the room to say goodbye. I cried as I held Josh's hand and touched the image of the baby's face and body on the screen. I said prayers and then told the little soul to go be with God and my other loved ones who have passed. I also said that we loved him or her and that we were so sorry.

The next day, the D&C went smoothly, and the doctors and nurses were wonderful. I didn't have much bleeding at first; however, a week or so later, right before Christmas, I did start bleeding more and having what felt like contractions. An ultrasound showed that the doctor didn't get all of the tissue during the D&C and that I might have to have a second D&C after the holidays. I was devastated and wanted this roller coaster ride of emotional and physical pain to be over.

Luckily, Christmas Eve, my body did what it was supposed to do and naturally rid the rest of the tissue. I was heartbroken and cried but felt relief that I wasn't going to need a second D&C. It was certainly a rough Christmas, but my inner faith, spirituality, and support system of family and friends were strong, and they helped Josh and I process all of the emotions.

TIP: Surround yourself with a good support system and network - family, friends, and various support groups.

That first loss came as such a shock to Josh and me because we already had a healthy child. We met later in life and married in 2013, when I was thirty-six and he was thirty-four. We had always wanted to become parents and both had loving childhoods growing up. We were excited to create our family.

We started trying for our first child in January of 2014. My OBGYN said, at my age, to try for six months, and then if nothing happened, she would refer me to a fertility specialist to get some basic testing done for Josh and me. She also checked my thyroid level, and though the results were normal, for optimal conception, they'd like to see the TSH level below 2.5. I started on the lowest dose of Levothyroxine to help get my numbers down. From then on, my thyroid levels were always monitored, especially during pregnancy.

TIP: Ask for an extended thyroid panel test.

At six months, we weren't pregnant, so I scheduled testing with a fertility specialist. We both had basic testing done, but there were certain tests that needed to be done on day two of my menstrual cycle. My cycle never started, but I kept getting negative pregnancy tests! I went in for a blood test to see what was going on and found I was just about to ovulate. Josh and I were perplexed but decided it was worth it for us to keep trying. If I didn't start my cycle in two weeks, the doctor would give me something to induce the start of my cycle.

We tried again and then left for a relaxing weekend trip. It was beautiful, and I completely forgot about trying to conceive. Two weeks later, we found out I was pregnant! I had a healthy pregnancy and gave birth to our precious son, Adam, in April of 2015, a couple weeks shy of my thirty-eighth birthday. We were happy we had a healthy baby and thrilled to become first-time parents.

TIP: Do basic fertility testing to help with a starting point.

We had wanted a two-year age difference between our children, and we were thrilled when we quickly got pregnant again in October of 2016.

Unfortunately, this was the pregnancy which led to that first shocking twelve-week miscarriage in December. It took us a while to heal from that first loss, but eventually, we were able to move forward with trying to conceive.

I turned forty in April of 2017, and Josh had switched jobs, so we had different insurance. I called our insurance company to see what was covered in terms of IVF or IUI. At first, the customer service representative was pleasant and told me I was covered for a few rounds of IVF and IUI. However, when she found out I was forty, she was hesitant and put me on hold to double check my coverage with her supervisor.

After almost ten minutes on hold, she bluntly told me that because I was over forty, our insurance only covered infertility testing and not any infertility treatment. She made me feel like being over forty was a disease, and I cried when I hung up. I felt so powerless and backed into a corner. I'm sure it was the stress of that news which caused the headaches a week later and, after two ER visits, eventually led to a shingles diagnosis on my head, face, and eye.

The shingles lasted what seemed like forever and was one of the most painful and debilitating experiences I have ever been through. I had to reach deep within myself spiritually to get through that initial pain and then the months of discomfort that followed. I had word stones that said "Faith" and "Believe" that I would hold in my hands to help me heal. I also experienced spiritual signs, such as seeing deer or hearing certain music and lyrics at various poignant moments, that kept me going.

I started doing acupuncture once a week since I had heard it could help with shingles. Josh and I were so relieved when the shingles healed. We were both in a space of gratitude that we had gone through so much and come out on the other side. We were happy to continue our fertility journey. The acupuncturist knew that we wanted to have a second child, so she started needling fertility points, which I believe helped me get pregnant again.

TIP: Seek out an acupuncturist that specializes in infertility.

We found out we were pregnant a few months later in November! I got the blood tests to confirm, and while my hCG numbers did double, the doctors felt like they were still a little low but hoped it was just because we tested early. They wanted to test me again after the Thanksgiving holiday. I certainly said many prayers over the next few days.

Josh, Adam, and I were out shopping when I got the call from the doctor with the results of my blood test. There in the car, in the Home Depot parking lot, it was confirmed; I was miscarrying at seven weeks. As Josh drove home, he held my hand while I silently cried. There were so many emotions. I was extremely discouraged, sad, and angry. What had happened? Why not this time? Why me? Why again? I had so many questions and no answers. The only answer was that I was having a second miscarriage.

Since the Christmas holiday was coming up, Josh and I decided to get a babysitter and have a much-needed night out for his holiday work party. We had a blast and forgot about all thing's fertility. I had always heard that a person can be more fertile after a miscarriage, and that was certainly true in our case. We found out a couple of weeks later, on December 28th, that we were expecting again! I called my OBGYN's office, and they said to come in after the holiday on

January 2nd to get my levels taken. Even though I felt fine physically, emotionally, I was scared that it wouldn't work out again.

After the holiday, the results from the tests were low and concerning. I knew in my heart that I was miscarrying. Hoping it wasn't true, I decided to take a pregnancy test again. It was negative. The same brand test that was positive just six days earlier. Then, within an hour, I started to bleed. This loss was fast and disappointing. That's when I learned what those early losses are called: chemical pregnancies. Why could I get pregnant but not stay pregnant?

I wanted answers. I wanted to find out if there was anything I could do to be proactive. I wanted to connect with others who were going through the same journey as I was. I joined an Over 40 and Trying to Conceive/Pregnancy Facebook group online. It was an amazing, helpful, and supportive resource. I started to read posts, learn from others' stories, and get support from people just like myself ... women not wanting to give up hope!

Josh and I decided to meet with a reproductive endocrinologist (RE) in Boston who had knowledge about couples experiencing multiple miscarriages. After a wonderful consultation, he scheduled more extensive testing for both of us. We were eager to know if there was a specific diagnosis that was causing these miscarriages.

TIP: If there is a need, get more extensive testing completed. In addition to further blood testing for genetics and hormone levels, we received these tests:

    a.   *Sperm count and motility tested again as well as a DNA sample from the sperm*

    b.   *Vaginal/pelvic ultrasound with follicle count*

    c.   *SIS: saline infusion sonography*
    d.   *Endometrial biopsy*

After the testing concluded, Josh and I met with the RE to discuss the results. We were happy yet baffled to find out that nothing was wrong. We left the office with mixed emotions and a sense of urgency because I was over forty. We took some deep breaths, and after talking about it, we decided to push that pressure aside and just keep focused on trying to conceive.

The next time we found out I was pregnant; I was about to have minor breast surgery to remove some atypical cells that could eventually turn into something more serious. When we found out I was pregnant, we had to postpone the surgery. My first HCG and progesterone levels came back pretty low, but it was still early. When we got the levels back from the second blood draw, we discovered that, unfortunately, it was not a viable pregnancy. I only knew I was pregnant for five days, but it was a crushing setback to my faith and hope.

I had developed a way to heal and move forward after each loss, so I could have a sense of closure. I would sit at my laptop with a box of tissues, listen to music, cry, and write our story. I would truly take the time to process what had happened, and it was my way of saying goodbye to these precious souls. I wrote about the amazing news of discovering I was pregnant, and about all the special, spiritual moments that came to me in words, songs, and signs. I printed out whatever tribute I wrote and put it in an envelope to file. I kept it with some memorabilia (like a Christmas card announcement that I never got to send or an ultrasound picture). This process helped me to focus, and feel positive about continuing our fertility journey.

TIP: If you experience a miscarriage, find a healthy way to get closure so that you can continue to heal and move forward.

My hope was dwindling. We felt defeated and discriminated against because of our age. At one point, the fertility doctor had mentioned that the odds were slim for us and that we should "just be happy with the child we have." Though that negative comment stung, we still felt he was a good doctor that we trusted. Since fertility testing was covered by our insurance, we had testing done multiple times, and the answer kept coming back the same: "You're both fine. Everything looks good but because you are older, the miscarriage rate is much higher – 50%." With IVF and IUI not an option for us because of cost, we just had to keep trying naturally.

I made peace with the fact that if we weren't successful, we would be a wonderful family of three. Voicing that out loud took a while, but once I did, I felt free and not so reliant on the outcome. I had a healthy dose of hope, faith, and belief that it *would* happen. I felt we weren't done with our journey yet and trusted that whatever was meant to happen would happen.

Despite everything we had been through, in December of 2018, between the loss and breast surgery, I think the dawning of the new year and my involvement in the Facebook group really helped change my attitude. I felt determined and confident as I did my daily positive affirmations in the mirror. I was choosing positivity and believing that there was a reason for all of this; a healthy little soul would come to us soon.

TIP: Make mental health a priority as a positive mindset is truly important.

This new positive attitude led me to make a few changes. I decided to try different supplements for a few months to see if it could help. I spoke with my doctor first, and though he said nothing is proven, it couldn't hurt. I also switched my ovulation tracking method. I had been using digital ovulation tests, which had become frustrating. I switched to the Easy at Home Ovulation Test Kit. I decided to treat it like a low stress science experiment and kept a log with all the results. It was interesting to see when I would get the peak every month.

> *TIP: The supplements I took were (please consult your doctor before taking any supplements or medication):*

    a.   *Prenatal vitamin with folic acid*
    b.   *Methyl folate*
    c.   *Vitamin D*
    d.   *Vitamin E*
    e.   *Low dose aspirin*
    f.   *Ubiquinol*

I could hardly believe my eyes when I got a positive pregnancy test just three months after I switched tracking methods and six months after the change in supplements! I called the OBGYN's office, and they immediately started me on progesterone. I was thrilled and in shock, praying this pregnancy would stick.

> *TIP: Ask your doctor about taking progesterone.*

I took each milestone during that pregnancy one at a time. I allowed myself to celebrate each milestone for a day and then slip back into "cautiously optimistic mode." Since I was forty-two, the entire pregnancy was monitored very closely, including an extra ultrasound that I requested at around ten weeks. We were excited to learn that the baby continued to grow and the heartbeat was strong.

We later found out we were having a girl, and all of the genetic testing looked good! We were excited yet nervous as the due date neared. Adam was curious about my growing belly and eager to meet his little sister.

Due to my age, the doctors didn't want me to deliver past my due date of February 12th, and, therefore, we had scheduled an induction for February 10th. My girl had other plans, though, and showed her beautiful head a few days early. Our rainbow baby girl, Emily, was born. I'm so proud that I was able to push out a nine-pound, three-ounce baby girl (with an epidural). Women are strong!

We now have a six-year-old and an eighteen-month-old who are blessings! We had wanted a smaller age difference, but in hindsight, it worked out perfectly. Adam is so sweet and helpful with Emily, and they just adore each other. We still look at Emily sometimes, amazed and grateful that, after all we went through, she finally came! Our family and my fertility journey were complete!

My first loss took my innocence regarding the process of conceiving, but the knowledge and the strength I gained far outweighs my losses. I learned so much about patience and perseverance. I remained positive yet practical and just kept *advocating* for myself, even at the doctor's office. I never gave up hope, especially when so many spiritual signs kept showing up.

I know miscarriage is common, but it's rarely brought to light as it's a sad and difficult experience to go through. I want to share our journey of hope because it is possible *and wonderful* to have a baby over the age of forty! After our bout with secondary infertility, the painful moments have faded, and the positive memories are stronger.

Nothing will top the moments our two adorable children entered this world!

TIP: Keep hope, have faith, and believe!

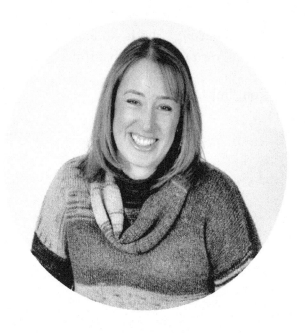

Scan the code for a video message from Diane and a free gift.

Diane (Moss) Prunier began her career in the entertainment industry after receiving a BFA in film and television production from Chapman University. During her 12 years in Los Angeles, she held various positions behind-the-scenes, including production coordinator for the CBS daytime show, "The Bold and the Beautiful."

Diane moved back to the east coast to become a certified professional life coach, starting her own business, Positive Pathways Coaching.

Though Diane is currently busy being a full-time mom, she does have a gift in mediumship. She is honing her skill to eventually branch out with her own mediumship business. Stay tuned!

dianeprunier.com/links

TO HELL AND BACK: A JOURNEY TO MOTHERHOOD

Susan Tozer

"I'm going to tell you something that
is going to blow your mind."

hose words still haunt me. Whenever I hear the words "blow your mind," I am taken back to that day in Dr. V.'s office. The 10th of December, 2009, the day our dream of starting a family shattered into a million sharp, heart-piercing pieces.

After my husband and I got married in October, 2001, at the age of 24, we decided to wait before starting a family. We were young and wanted to see the world. If only we knew how precious those years would prove to be. At age 27, we decided we might be ready to start a family. Our mindset was that if it happens, it happens. At that stage, I was very naïve and ignorant about fertility. We stopped all contraception and started "making babies."

We were ecstatic to find out at Christmas 2006 that we were pregnant, two years after we had stopped contraception. I never thought to do the math because we were in no hurry to conceive. We were living in England at the time and travelling Europe._

> *Tip: Consider seeking help to conceive if you are younger than 35 and have been trying to conceive for at least a year or if you're 35 or older and have been trying to conceive for at least 6 months. Seek help from a medical professional specializing in fertility. Do not hesitate to go for second or third opinions.*

Throughout my twenties, I only had regular periods while I was taking oral contraceptives. Without them, my periods were erratic and varied in length. I never knew when to expect it.

At the end of January, 2007, our world fell apart for the first time when I had a miscarriage. We were about ten weeks along. We nicknamed the baby "Beanie" early in the pregnancy, and that is what we have always called him. I say 'him' because, in my heart, I have always thought of him as a boy.

We heard the usual ignorant comments like "at least it happened early," "hopefully the next one sticks," "you're still young; you can try again," "there was obviously something wrong with it." 'It' was our baby, and we didn't want a different baby. We already loved him.

Now what? Do we just wake up the next morning and continue with our lives as if nothing had happened? No funeral? No flowers or sympathy cards?

I gritted my teeth, tried to push the feelings down, and got on with life. "There was hardly a baby there. Stop feeling sorry for yourself. Other people have gone through much worse," I'd tell myself.

> *Tip: Allow yourself time to grieve a loss. Seek counseling or at least a supportive, understanding person to speak to. Ignoring the emotions or blaming yourself delays healing.*

I thought I had done something to cause the miscarriage. I thought perhaps I wasn't meant to be a mother, that maybe I wouldn't be a good enough mother. Deep down, I knew there was something wrong with my body. I had a gut feeling for a long time. Something wasn't right.

Over the next two years, I wasted many hours seeing doctors who thought they knew about fertility. They dismissed me and told me nothing was wrong. "Make an appointment for blood tests on the second day of your next period," they'd suggest. How? With these erratic periods, I don't know when the second day will be. "You don't ovulate regularly. Just make sure you have intercourse every second day." Sounds easy, doesn't it? Sounds like fun, doesn't it? It made me feel like we weren't trying hard enough. Maybe we were "doing it" wrong.

The lab messed up my husband's sperm analysis results and wrote in large, red letters "LOW MOTILITY." Dr. V. would later discard that piece of paper with the remark, "Based on what?!" It turned out; my husband's swimmers were perfectly fine.

I believed all the ridiculous things people say. "Relax, you're thinking about it too much." "If you go on holiday/move house/get a new job/pray harder, you will fall pregnant." I tried all those things. In the meantime, my friends were having their first or second children.

Back home in South Africa, in June, 2009, we decided it was time to seek help from a fertility specialist.

The fertility clinic did a full work up on both of us. At the initial scan, Dr. V. shook his head and said, "These ovaries are very quiet." I didn't know what that meant. I do now.

While waiting for the test results, I thought they would tell me I'd need to use the drug Clomid, which I had heard helped so many friends of my friends fall pregnant. Worst case scenario, I thought we'd have to do IVF. I spent time reading up a lot on fertility treatments, joined an online forum for women struggling to conceive, and somewhere along the way, I read an article on women making use of egg donors. "How wonderful," I thought. "Perhaps I'll donate some of my eggs once we've had our babies."

One day in December, 2009, Dr. V. called and requested to see us immediately. I knew then that something was very wrong. I got some numbers out of him on the phone, entered it into a search engine online, found an article, sank down onto my knees, and started sobbing. Please, no. Please, God, don't do this to us. Thankfully, I was working at home. I hoped that I had misunderstood what I had read. We went to see Dr. V. the next day. He entered the office, and in his soft-spoken, serious manner, said, "I'm going to tell you something that is going to blow your mind."

What I had read online was true. I was 32 years old, had hardly any eggs left, and those I did have were of terrible quality. It's called premature ovarian failure (POF). I had a very high FSH (follicle-stimulating hormone) level, nearly undetectable AMH (anti-Müllerian hormone) level, and very low antral follicle count. Dr. V. told us that our chances of conceiving naturally were extremely low, and if successful, chances of miscarriage were quite high. I had "the ovaries of a fifty-year-old." He said that, of course, it's not impossible that we could conceive naturally and carry a healthy baby to term, and should this happen, he would be the first to congratulate us.

> *Tip: Premature ovarian failure (POF), also known as primary ovarian insufficiency (POI), is a loss of ovarian function before the age of 40. POF can affect women from their teenage years to their thirties. Women with POF are at a greater risk of a range of health issues, including osteoporosis, estrogen deficiency, and heart diseases. The loss of ovarian function means that the probability of a woman falling pregnant with her own eggs is greatly reduced.*

Dr. V. told us the best chance we had of conceiving and carrying a baby to term was using donor eggs (DE). He explained that I could expect to go into menopause early. It was a massive shock. I tried to ask questions between sobs. My husband was stunned and trying to make sense of exactly what we were up against. He asked whether it would be worth trying an IVF cycle with my eggs. Dr. V. responded that we could try, of course, but that the cycle could be cancelled because I wouldn't respond well enough to the medication. He said that he wouldn't, in good conscience, suggest an IVF cycle with my eggs and take our money.

I couldn't understand how this could be possible. Was it something I did? Was I being punished by God for something? I couldn't think of anything I could have done that could possibly warrant this punishment and pain. Rapists, pedophiles, and murderers get to have children. Even flies have babies!

We were devastated. My husband cried and said, "I don't want another woman's babies. I want your babies." My heart broke again at that. I had to go through a grieving process and a lot of therapy to come to terms with the idea of using another woman's eggs and my potential child not having my genes. Would I be able to bond with this child? Would they one day reject me as not being their "real mom"? I was ashamed and embarrassed. I felt like I wasn't a real woman. I offered to help my husband find a better, proper, fertile wife. He wasn't impressed with that suggestion at all. I hated my body. I hated myself. I was broken, less than, old, barren.

We looked for a donor that had the same physical features as me, someone we felt a connection with while reading her profile. It felt weird, like shopping for an egg carrier. In South Africa, egg donation is anonymous – unless you use a family member or friend who offers to donate her eggs. I armed myself with information and made learning everything I could about this condition and process my new mission in life.

> *Tip: Everyone has different things they look for in a donor profile. What helped me was to imagine myself writing a donor profile. Would someone pick me? It is not possible to find a perfect, cardboard cut-out woman.*

We jumped in and then … that first DE IVF attempt didn't work.

This was 2010. We went through this process another six times with another five donors.

Read donor profiles. Choose a donor. Wait for a period to start. Start oral contraceptives – because that's how we get pregnant. Wait for the donor to start her period and take all her meds. Go for scans. Pray. Beg. Cry. Hope. Wait for news on the egg retrieval. Wait for the fertilization report. Wait for day 5. Another embryo transfer. Another excruciating two week wait. Another negative pregnancy test. More tears. More screaming into a pillow in rage. Lots of therapy. Perfecting a fake smile. Picking myself up off the floor. Putting one foot in front of the other. Working hard to earn money for the next attempt. Lots of wine. Rinse and repeat.

With each attempt, we'd tweak something. Slightly different meds, ZIFT (zygote intrafallopian transfer), intralipids, and so on. There was no explanation as to why it wasn't working. There seemed to be nothing else wrong with my body. After the ZIFT, Dr. V. confirmed that my ovaries looked like raisins.

My husband would read donor profiles and make spreadsheets for me, listing the characteristics of each donor. I would then make a shortlist and read those profiles before we decided on one together.

Along the way, donors we had selected were rejected for hereditary conditions, concerns over hormone levels, and dishonesty. I could try to describe every attempt, but it all became a bit of a blur, and the worst was yet to come.

Tip: Arm yourself with as much information as you can. Take questions and a notepad along to consultations. It is often a lot of information to take in.

I hated it when people said that it would "happen in God's time." If someone would just tell me when that time would be, then I could get on with my life until that time arrived. I hated that four-letter word 'just.' 'Just' adopt, 'just' use a surrogate, 'just' relax.

At some point, Dr. V. mentioned surrogacy. We went to a presentation on surrogacy with an open mind but decided against it. Everyone has a line, and that was ours. I couldn't face watching another woman carry my baby.

The final suggestion Dr. V. made was regression therapy because, as he conveyed to me in an email: "I believe there are deeper issues, issues that neither you, me nor Raymond are aware of, that inhibit conception and prevent us from having the outcome that we want. Quantum physics literature is clear on the fact that 'if the vessel is not 100% sound', meaning not just physically, but at a deeply emotional level, that nothing positive will happen in that vessel, but that a spiral will start that will continue to spiral downwards until the issue/s are resolved. There are countless examples of couples not being able to conceive due to *a deep-seated emotional issue* that prevents this from happening. I believe this may be the case in your instance."

He referred me to a clinical psychologist specializing in regression therapy via hypnosis, Dr. O. We were very surprised and a little skeptical about this. Until then, we hadn't met a medical professional that had a holistic perspective. We decided to trust Dr. V. since we didn't have another plan anyway.

And so, in 2012, I started down a path straight through hell, a path that would change me forever and, after which, I'd need therapy for many years to come.

> *Tip: Therapy to deal with trauma is invaluable. There is great benefit in having someone that is not emotionally involved help you to process the feelings around the trauma that you suffered, regardless of how 'big' the trauma was.*

Hypnotherapy is not what you might have seen on television, where a person is made to cluck like a chicken, apparently without knowing what they're doing. I can describe it as what happens when you're driving a car, deep inside a memory, not completely focusing on the road, and suddenly, a dog runs in front of your car. Immediately, you are back to the present time, slamming your foot down on the brake. You were present, yet not quite.

I went into the process thinking that, deep down, I believed that I wouldn't be a good enough mother or that I didn't deserve to be a mother. There were some sessions during which it felt like we hardly made any progress. We started off exploring my childhood, my birth, my parenting, and at some point, Dr. O. asked me to visualize what my womb looks like. I saw a black, sludgy pool bubbling with poison. We had to discover why it looked like that. Through a few hellish sessions, I discovered that I had been repeatedly sexually abused by a family member that used to babysit me. In the worst incident, I heard what I can only describe as my soul screaming. It was incredibly traumatic. I remember thinking, at the time, that this must be what hell feels like. I often wanted to give up, but I needed to see this through if I was to heal and fulfill our dream of having a child.

Next, I had to, under hypnosis, fix the damage to my womb, to clean out all the poison. By the middle of 2013, I felt healed enough to continue with the next DE IVF cycle.

The monster that abused me died at the end of 2013. That little girl was now free and safe at last.

Our last attempt with DE IVF was at the start of 2014. I was done looking for a donor. Done reading profiles. I insisted (i.e., asked very nicely) that the clinic find a donor for us. We couldn't care less what she looked like, so long as it worked. The only physical characteristics we had in common was our height and the shape of our noses. This was it. We had reached the end of our tether. In that last cycle, we did things differently. We decided to spend the two-week wait for the results on holiday at the coast rather than trying to stay busy at work. I like to joke that I went on holiday and came back pregnant, like everyone said I should do.

Our beautiful daughter was born in November, 2014, after a relatively easy pregnancy. She is feisty, assertive, strong-willed, and utterly adorable.

And you know what? It doesn't matter one iota to me that she doesn't have my genes. Genetics isn't what makes a family. If any of those other cycles had worked, we wouldn't have had this child. Yes, we might have had someone else, but not her, and we cannot imagine our life without her. I know we were meant to be together. Infertility and fertility treatment is no walk in the park, and it costs a fortune, but in the end, the journey was worth every cent we spent and every tear we shed.

We are forever grateful to our donor, whomever and wherever she is, for the enormous gift she has given us. She didn't just give us some eggs. She gave us a lifetime of memories and firsts. First birthday, first tooth, first laugh, first steps, first words, first "I love you, mommy," first tantrum, first day of school, and all the other normal things that parents experience.

Tip: Make self-care a priority. Not 'soft' self-care in the shape of candle-lit bubble baths, but 'messy' self-care in the form of being selective who you share information with, putting yourself first, and strong boundaries. Start cultivating healthy coping mechanisms and methods of stress relief. If possible, join a support group – in person or online. I found talk therapy to be invaluable. PPD and/ or PTSD is prevalent among infertile women using ART (assisted reproductive technology) to conceive.

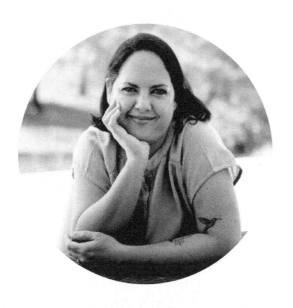

Scan the code for a video message from Susan and a free gift

Susan Tozer has lived a life that people write novels about. Now, she is taking pen to paper to do just that herself. From miscarriage to infertility and so much more, Susan brings her wit and charm to her brutally honest and refreshing stories.

By day, Susan works as a software developer and, in her spare time, can be found fighting dragons or catching unicorns with her much dreamed of daughter. Susan's other passion lies in helping infertile women like herself find solace and companionship and enlightening the public on infertility.

https://linktr.ee/susantozer

A SECOND CHANCE AT MOTHERHOOD

Brandi Bunda

grew up in a single-parent home with an incarcerated father, which brought about its own set of challenges and hardships. I was a typical little girl, playing house, pretending to be a mom, and caring for my life-like babies. I was naturally the nurturing type. I always knew I wanted to be a mom, but I never imagined it would happen at such a young age. Shockingly, I was in junior high when I became pregnant after having sex for the very first time. I was 14 years old.

Figuring out how to raise and financially support another human was scary, daunting, and, honestly, didn't seem possible. Without any support from my family, there was no way I could do it on my own, so my mom drove me to a clinic in a neighboring state, and I had an abortion. I was 12 weeks pregnant. I have a hole in my heart that only that baby can fill, and the pain, shame, and guilt still haunt me today.

I know my life would have been so different as a teen mom. Around the same time, I got to witness the struggle and sacrifice first-hand when one of my closest friends also became pregnant. She had the support of her family, went through with her pregnancy, and raised her baby. Walking that journey alongside her was a constant reminder of what I had done and the baby I didn't have.

I graduated high school with honors and headed off to college, where I met my husband. We dated for 5 years before getting married. Shortly after we got married in 2010, I embarked on somewhat of a wellness journey when I started working for a holistic supplement company in the animal health industry. I became inundated with learning about preventative health and natural wellness, for both pets and people.

After waiting a year and a half, we wanted to start a family, I was 29 at the time. So, I stopped taking birth control, ditched the Adderall, cut out soda, and started taking a prenatal vitamin daily.

Sadly, five months into my fertility journey, my dad got diagnosed with stage 4 lung cancer. I became his primary caregiver and together we made dietary and lifestyle changes to improve our health. We started buying more organic meats and veggies, choosing non-GMO products, eating less packaged food, and cutting down on processed sugar. We were more intentional with taking our supplements every day and were introduced to the world of essential oils and aromatherapy.

Surprisingly, two weeks after my dad finished his last day of treatment, we found out we were pregnant! We were ecstatic and over the moon with excitement! Having just gone through one of the toughest seasons of our entire lives, this news was such a blessing. We quickly made a doctor's appointment to get confirmation, and the day we heard the heartbeat for the very first time, I experienced a wave of unexplainable joy and gratitude. I thanked Jesus repeatedly for hearing and answering our prayers.

We went out to eat with some family members to celebrate, but our celebration was short-lived. Not long after getting home from the restaurant, I started cramping and passing small blood clots in our bathroom. I had never experienced a miscarriage before, so I was unsure if that's what was happening. I retrieved the clots from the toilet and we rushed to the hospital. After being admitted, an ultrasound confirmed there was no heartbeat. I was sent home to rest, get comfortable, and wait for my body to stop bleeding, which could take at least a week or more.

The thought of having a miscarriage *never* really crossed my mind. We were completely devastated and with broken hearts, we buried our baby under the old bodark tree, not far from our dog, Bit-Bit, who had passed away earlier that year. It was a sad and difficult time, to say the least.

If I'm being really honest, at that moment, I questioned whether I was even worthy of being a mom. Earlier in life, I had taken one precious life for granted, and now I was asking to be blessed with another. *Why? Why do I deserve to be a mom?* It brought up some deep-rooted emotions and took me back to being that scared junior high kid who had the opportunity to be a mom but had no other choice than to give it up.

I believe many girls or women who make a similar decision, for whatever reason, likely suffer silently in the aftermath, unaware of the far-reaching effects this decision will trigger in their lives, and struggle to believe that God could ever forgive them. I know this was true for me, but thankfully, where trauma inflicts devastating pain, God extends abundant love and grace.

I opened up to those closest to me, like my husband and my parents, sharing my fears, but I never said anything to anyone else. I often wondered if something happened during that procedure all those years ago that would prohibit me from having kids today. Fortunately, I had a strong and encouraging support system that loved me unconditionally, without judgment.

At a follow-up appointment, my OBGYN assured us that early miscarriage was completely normal and explained that many women experience a miscarriage more often than we realize because it's not something that is talked about enough.

She suggested I get my progesterone levels checked, so I popped into her office a few weeks later. My levels came back lower than normal. I immediately ordered a progesterone serum infused with vitamin E and essential oils. I applied it over my forearms and inner ankles morning and night to help increase my levels to sustain a healthy pregnancy.

TIP: Seek guidance from a coach or a mentor, so you don't walk this path alone. Feel empowered to take control of your fertility health from the very beginning.

I began to incorporate more and more essential oils and other supplements into my regimen for physical, mental, and emotional support. Despite this, I still had a plethora of symptoms like acne, mouth ulcers, excessive sweating, trouble sleeping, chronic headaches, hypoglycemia, anemia, fatigue, fainting episodes, tingling arms, bloating, abdominal cramps, neck, back, and joint pain, keratosis (tiny bumps/rash on my skin), and digestive issues like constipation and diarrhea.

I made several visits to my primary care doctor, and he suggested treatments such as Metamucil for my digestive issues, Ambien for sleep, and an NSAID for pain. He even scheduled an MRI to scan my brain to rule out a possible tumor that could be pressing on my pituitary gland, contributing to my chronic headaches, and causing an imbalance in hormone production. Gratefully, there were no significant abnormalities or tumors present. He also ordered a complete blood work-up, a comprehensive metabolic panel, and checked my iron levels and thyroid function. All came back relatively *normal*. But my symptoms persisted.

Unsure of what to do next, I spent the entire year of 2013 being more intentional about my health on a quest to get to the root of my issues.

I made frequent trips to the chiropractor, continued to track my cycle and basal temperature each month, bought over-the-counter ovulation kits, and even arranged my work travel schedule (covering 5 states) around my most fertile window. During that time, sex was both scheduled and spontaneous. We tried all the recommended tips, changing time of day, positions, and even relaxing with my feet up and pelvis elevated for half an hour after intercourse. I did all the things Dr. Google recommends! I even stood on my head one time for like 20 minutes (*no joke, I felt desperate!*)

I did not have a typical 28-day cycle. My periods were so irregular, I was *late* nearly every month, which is a total mind f* when you are trying to have a baby! As a result, I took a LOT of pregnancy tests.

> *TIP: Incorporate essential oils labeled for topical use and aromatherapy into your daily regimen. Find healthy ways to reduce stress and manage emotions (write in a gratitude journal daily + journal your feelings as often as you feel led).*

By textbook standards, there didn't seem to be anything *wrong* with me. I never had an abnormal pap smear, nor did I suffer from PCOS or endometriosis. I didn't have an issue ovulating and had gotten pregnant once before, so that was a plus in the eyes of my OB. The next step was to refer me to a fertility specialist, but I was hesitant and uninterested at the time. I had a strong desire to pursue pregnancy naturally, without medical intervention.

Nearly two years into my fertility journey, I was traveling out of state for work when a conversation with a co-worker led to a discussion about gut health and the possibility of food triggers contributing to my digestive issues. I often looked like I was 4-5 months pregnant, constantly bloated, and achy with irritated skin. I started doing research online from my phone and was convinced I had celiac disease.

As soon as I got home, I scheduled an appointment with my primary care doctor for blood work. A week later, my results came back and my numbers were within the *normal range*. They confirmed I **didn't** have celiac disease and advised me that there was no need to restrict gluten from my diet, so I didn't.

> *TIP: Find a functional, integrative or naturopathic doctor to help run preconception and micronutrient tests. Iron, hormones, thyroid, MTHFR, food sensitivities*

I wanted to see if improving my gut health would improve my fertility, so I looked into local naturopathic doctors in my area. That's when I found Dr. M. She was extremely busy with an 8-week waiting list for new patients, but I made my appointment anyway.

While I waited, my sister-in-law recommended a nutrition advisor who performed health and longevity scans using biocommunication software. In December 2013, I booked an appointment with a lady who conducted what's called a ZYTO scan, which provided information to help me make individual wellness choices using galvanic skin response technology. The results of my scan analysis suggested I needed support in the following areas: antioxidants, B-vitamins, enzymes, essential fatty acids, gut microbes, and good bacteria, minerals, and vitamin D, as well as endocrine and hormonal support for the adrenals and the thyroid.

I was blown away by the information I received. I didn't quite understand how the software worked, but I was willing to look into all the recommendations. This particular report also suggested various products that could be easily incorporated into my daily wellness regimen.

In January 2014, I attended a 48-day transformation seminar with my dad, hosted by the naturopath I was going to see the following month. It was super informative and left me eager for our appointment. I can honestly say that this was the beginning of an incredibly transformative time for me. Dr. M. legitimately changed my life.

Our first visit was 3 hours long! She asked me health questions as far back as my mom's pregnancy, my infancy, if I was breast or formula-fed, if I was sickly growing up, what immunizations I had been exposed to, any surgeries I had, medications or antibiotics I'd been prescribed, and my entire health history up until that very moment. We discussed all my symptoms and my current regimen.

During our initial visit, she conducted several tests, including a food sensitivity test. Surprisingly, I had a *negative response* to barley, gluten, wheat, and rye. I couldn't believe it. I was surprised and confused. My primary care doctor said I could eat gluten, yet this food sensitivity test indicated otherwise. This is when I learned how food sensitivities and intolerances directly contribute to an immune response in the body that can cause leaky gut or intestinal permeability, which then leads to chronic inflammation, mineral and nutrient deficiencies, and hormonal imbalances -- all contributing factors to infertility.

Dr. M. requested I start an elimination diet to remove my food triggers, follow the paleo diet, focus on healing my body, and wait 6 months before actively trying to conceive. This would give me the greatest chance of sustaining a healthy pregnancy.

I learned that there is a direct correlation between gut health, the endocrine system, and hormone production. We discussed various ways I could support my hormones while eliminating toxic products from my home that have a cumulative and negative effect on the body. She suspected I was also suffering from severe adrenal fatigue, and my coffee habit was a contributing factor, so she nixed my daily cup of joe while we worked to heal my body holistically.

TIP: Begin an elimination diet to improve nutrition, reduce chronic inflammation, and start the process of healing your gut. Use quality supplements, including probiotics and digestive enzymes, and know which prenatal is best for your body.

Although the thought of keeping a food journal seemed daunting, something changed in me that day. I felt more in control of my health. I was optimistic about my future. Now, I had options and a game plan, whereas before, my only next step was medical intervention with a fertility specialist. By the time I left Dr. M.'s office, I was inspired and empowered to make these dietary and lifestyle changes in hopes that it would get me closer to having the family I'd been praying for.

I immediately cut out coffee, gluten, and sugar and started following the paleo diet, which closely resembles the autoimmune protocol (AIP) diet. I changed up the supplements I was taking every day. I continued to use essential oils for mental, physical, and emotional support, and I started ditching the toxic products I was using in my home that was no longer serving me, including my beloved scented candles and air fresheners.

> *TIP: Slowly detox your home from toxic household and personal care products that inhibit your endocrine and reproductive systems' ability to perform and function at their best. Ditching products with synthetic fragrances, such as candles, perfumes, and conventional household cleaners, is an easy place to start.*

Two months after my initial appointment with Dr. M., we got the news that my dad was cancer-free. It seemed unbelievable that 18 months after he was released from conventional treatment because the doctors could no longer help him, we beat this battle on our own. *But we did.* What a blessing! Thank you, Jesus!

For me, it was proof that our bodies were designed for miraculous healing, and it gave me the hope and motivation to stay the course. I used an app on my phone to keep track of my cycles and when I was ovulating, but I kept in mind Dr. M.'s request to give her six months before actively trying to conceive. I honored my body, focused on improving my health, and spent less time worrying about getting pregnant, which is not easy in the least.

Over time, I felt so much better physically, mentally, and emotionally, and my symptoms slowly started to subside. My acne went away, the keratosis disappeared, my chronic headaches diminished, I wasn't bloated, I had regular bowel movements, I had seemingly less stress and tons of energy, and surprisingly, my periods were on a predictable 28-day cycle for the first time in years. I couldn't believe it!

It was Labor Day weekend when I found myself sitting alone at church for the first time in a long time. I felt so moved by the message that, with tears in my eyes, a lump in my throat, and chills all over my body, I raised my hand and recommitted my life to Christ. I made plans to get baptized the following month alongside my dad, who had never been baptized before. It was such a special and memorable moment.

Less than 2 weeks after that, I was *late* for the first time in months.

It was a little unusual since I was finally regulating my cycle. "I ran to the store for pregnancy tests. I took the first one and waited. I saw two blue lines. I immediately took another test and waited. Again, there were two blue lines. I was shocked, surprised, and speechless. I made an appointment with my OBGYN for the following week, and she confirmed." We were PREGNANT!

We were ecstatic but hesitant to celebrate. We waited until Thanksgiving before we shared the news with our family.

I stayed intentional with all the changes I had made, hired a midwife, went to breastfeeding and birthing classes, incorporated prenatal massage, and went on to have a wonderfully healthy pregnancy. I felt very passionate about natural childbirth, so I was determined to have my baby without the use of medications or an epidural. Two weeks before my daughter's due date, our perfect little firecracker made her grand entrance, on Independence Day of all days!

TIP: Hire a midwife or a doula if you are seeking natural childbirth. Eat protein first thing in the morning to help

> *avoid nausea + morning sickness. Encapsulate your placenta to help improve milk supply and mood and decrease chances for postpartum depression.*

Nothing can replace the feeling of holding our baby for the first time and looking into her big, brown eyes. I'd say struggling with infertility made me a better mom. The positive changes I made followed me into motherhood, trickled into the way I parent, and enlightened my perspective about the ability of our bodies.

Interestingly, I was in the process of weaning my daughter from breastfeeding at 28 months postpartum when we found out we were PREGNANT again! At our ultrasound, we were nearly 16 weeks along. This time, it happened without all the heartache, constant struggle, and years of trying and failing. I'm so grateful for my beautiful gifts of life and feel deeply inspired to help others on their journey to motherhood.

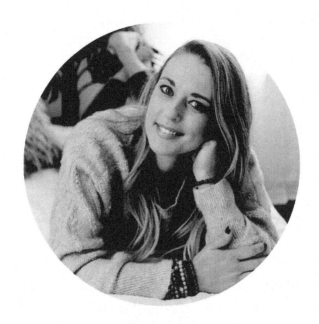

Scan the code for a video message from Brandi and a free gift

Brandi Bunda is a health and wellness coach with a heart for helping women navigate their fertility journey while on their way to becoming a mom. Having survived unexplained infertility, she is super passionate about teaching others how to integrate functional medicine practices into their daily wellness and encouraging a holistic approach to helping women get pregnant naturally.

If you are ready to search for the root cause of your infertility and want to optimize your chances of staying pregnant, then you are in the right place, and Brandi is here to help support, encourage, and guide you!

https://brandibunda.com/page/links?fbclid=IwAR1ti_dAh5D7Ng4j42QJ7pAn6Xm3ktVQSTt6l6MQ2M7n1pa6_8NiHs38Vks

INFERTILITY: MY UNEXPECTED BLESSING

Cindy Grace

I can remember it like it was yesterday; we got married and went on our honeymoon, and a month and a half later, I received some of the happiest news of my life. I was pregnant! Oh my gosh, it was so fast but such a blessing!

However, in a blink of an eye, that same great news taught me that not all blessings last forever. Real blessings may come from events out of our control. Real blessings may even push us so far out of our comfort zones that it is hard for us to even recognize the face we see in the mirror. That was me.

Fast forward to the six-week mark of my pregnancy, and my little controlled environment of newlywed bliss was about to be a mere shell of what it was just weeks prior. I began to feel cramping and pain, and I was concerned. Then, the reality of the word "blessing" hit me, and it was pain and heartache that I had never felt before.

My blood levels were off, and the doctor's concern for the viability of the pregnancy were heightened. As each week passed, I was more terrified, and it was the kind of fear that changes you. You want to control everything around you, but you can't. Then, my worst nightmare happened. I lost that little blessing faster than I could have ever imagined. That miscarriage is when the trajectory of my motherhood journey drastically changed forever.

After I mourned the very unexpected loss of our baby, I visited my first infertility specialist and quickly found out that my miscarriage was not a fluke. Though, on paper, I looked like the ideal candidate for a successful pregnancy, something was off because I could not get pregnant again. When I met with the doctor, he placed me on a round of Clomid. I have to be honest; I thought I would take some Clomid and get pregnant a couple of months later. However, that was definitely not the case.

Needless to say, both attempts at Clomid failed, and we proceeded to intrauterine insemination (IUI). We had another round of failures, and I am the one that pulled the plug on more IUIs and asked to go straight to in vitro fertilization (IVF). Remember that loss of control I spoke about earlier? Calling the shots was the way I was taking the control back, and my IVF journey began.

Tip: Ask the doctor the best- and worst-case scenarios for every medication and procedure, so you are fully informed if the procedure is right for your specific fertility struggles.

I have to admit, my first IVF procedure terrified me. A journey like infertility is the perfect storm of feeling inadequate mixed with feeling at fault. I started my birth control to regulate my cycle for retrieval, and I poked myself with almost every needle in the package, made myself bleed, bruised myself, felt a roller coaster of hormonal emotions, and was unable to sit comfortably for days.

Ultrasound after ultrasound, everything was stimulating well, eggs were forming and maturing, and the retrieval was on schedule. I looked like I had about 12 mature eggs. I arrived for retrieval, and I was in such good spirits because it all went so well, until it didn't.

I went home, hyper stimulated, and then got the call no one ever wants. There were only two viable eggs, and though they both fertilized, only one looked promising.

I am sure you can guess the rest of the story. I had the one embryo transferred, and it failed. I remember seeing my children in my dreams, feeling the happiness and the warmth of their love wrapped in my arms like it was happening in real life. I decided to try again with another round of IVF, but this time, I was going to take matters into my own hands. I changed my diet, I went to acupuncture, I took more supplements than I could count, I did fertility yoga, and I listened to fertility meditations; incidentally, both the yoga and the fertility meditation helped immensely for a variety of reasons, which I explain in my blog.

Tip: Take time for yourself. Fertility yoga, fertility meditations supplements, and treating yourself with abundant grace and kindness all help the process.

God bless my persistent heart, my second round of IVF failed, too. Then, it happened. The doctor looked me right in my face and told me I would most likely never have children. *How could this be?* My entire family was fertile beyond their means.

This could not be how my story ends. Unlike most other women struggling with infertility, my doctor gave me no reason why I could not get pregnant. This made researching a specialist nearly impossible. I spent countless hours researching, and with an immense amount of prayer, I found the one doctor who would soon be my next blessing. This doctor had success rates I never thought possible.

Do you want to know something? Good doctors report their success rates. Want to know something else? My original doctor never did!

I met with my new doctor, and he quickly told me there was nothing in my testing that would indicate that I could not have children. I was shocked, hopeful, hesitant, and a little angry all rolled into one.

You know the drill -- needle after needle, med after med, supplement after supplement, fertility yoga, mindset work, you name it, I did it. Soon, I was back in the office for retrieval.

This doctor had explained to me that most patients do not know that the standard of a clinic's equipment and staff matter. I was so happy they were able to show me why their equipment was leaps and bounds better than my last doctor's and why that improved my odds immensely.

Tip: The level of equipment in the facility, the skill of the embryo handlers, the success rates of the doctor, etc., all play a substantial role in the success of the IVF cycle.

Well, by this time, you may have guessed it; with the help of my new specialist, there I was after my third fresh IVF cycle, getting the call I had only dreamt of. I remember the very moment. Time stopped, my breath stopped, and she said the words, *"Cindy, you're pregnant, and your HCG levels look amazing."* I fell to my knees and began to sob. I thanked her and immediately started running around my living room screaming, "OH MY GOD, OH MY GOD, OH MY GOD!"

I then started thinking about how I was going to tell my husband and my parents. After telling my husband and taking the excitement in, I had to wait until the dreaded week number six, when I had found out my first baby would most likely not make it. This wait was going to be a painful one, but there was no way around it.

The six-week appointment came. Lying there, I could not see the monitor; only my husband and the doctor could. There was agonizing DEAD SILENCE. In my mind, I am saying, "Yep, I knew it, no baby, or the baby has no heartbeat, and they don't have the heart to tell me."

Finally, I shout out, "UMMMM, HELLO, anyone? Anyone want to tell me what is happening?"

The doctor pauses, and I hear, "Well, Cindy, I have some news for you."

The next words forever changed my life in so many ways. The doctor said, "We definitely have a heartbeat; in fact, we have two." TWO? "Yes, you are having twins."

Now, I knew they put in two embryos, but they also put in two embryos with both of my failed IVF cycles. This time, both embryos stuck, and their hearts were beating strongly. I looked at my husband, who looked a mixture of "Dear Jesus, help me" and "I better look excited or this woman, who just put herself through emotional and physical hell, may kill me."

Two babies? Two sets of everything! Two strollers, two cribs … I could not be happier; I was a twin mom! With all of that complete happiness, you would think the pain from the struggle to get to this day would disappear, but can I be totally transparent with you? A journey like that changes you … forever. You are never truly who you once were, and that spills over onto so many aspects of the future.

A few years after my twin boys were born, I knew I wanted another baby. I was actually able to freeze the third embryo from the boys' fresh cycle. It should be a no-brainer, right? My body had been through a full pregnancy.

To make a long story short, that was not what happened, and that frozen embryo failed. I thought I would not try again after that, but once I had that third baby in my mind and the love I had for my other two children, I knew I had to try again.

I proceeded to go through three more fresh IVF cycles and two more frozen cycles before the final miracle of my daughter arrived three years after her brothers. Yep! You read that right -- five additional cycles for a whopping total of eight IVF cycles in all. Today, I have three of the most beautiful, funny, intelligent, and talented children on this earth, and I thank the Lord Jesus Christ for giving me the strength to stay his course in order to bring them earthside.

With that being said, I am also recovering. I'm recovering from the loss of my very first child, recovering from going through a three-year journey that will forever impact who I am today and the mother I was going to be.

As mothers already know, motherhood is one perpetual rollercoaster ride that has the highest highs and the lowest lows and can often make you feel like you are living in fight or flight mode. I am the happiest I have ever been in my life, but at times, I still feel waves of uncertainty in different aspects of my life.

On the flip side, my journey has also shown me the strength, endurance, perseverance, and beauty of my own human person. Your journey writes portions of the story of your life, but can illustrate the rest of your story the way you want, which is what I gradually began to do.

For me, these past patterns of unbalance, uneasiness, and uncontrolled outcomes began to manifest themselves in a need to control and prove my worth. I was never going to feel that feeling of failure again. I was never going to have that feeling of derailment, uncertainty, mistrust, and vulnerability.

I knew I wanted to be the best mother I could ever be, giving my children everything and anything within my reach. To be honest, even if it wasn't in my reach, my kids would have anything I deemed necessary for their happiness. This ensured that I avoided reliving all of my past fears, but it also took every ounce of energy I had to live in that manner.

Knowing in my heart that I could never truly control my way out of that fear again, and that my potential for reliving that same feeling of defeat was most likely inevitable, I continued to fill every minute of my day with what I thought it meant to be a good mother. I tried to "balance" my friendships, marriage, work schedule, and my children's growth and happiness, feeding them healthy meals and supplements and ensuring they had proper sleep, all while inwardly feeling unraveled.

My house looked like a disaster, I was nursing (so difficult, yet so worth it), and sleep was something I had forgotten existed, but these children were my life, and I was going to be present and give them all of me, even if it killed me.

Finally, I had to have a come-to-Jesus with myself. I had to tell myself that this "successful" lifestyle was nothing short of chaos and overwhelm, and if, God forbid, I experienced the same trauma I did throughout my infertility journey, then, so be it because this was not what happiness was all about.

Give it all to God Cindy and you work on you. Man, my head was spinning because this was going to take even more strength and courage, but I knew I was going to have to make myself a priority *the same way* I prioritized fighting to have my kids.

I had taken a journey of 1,000 women, and I fought and traveled that journey over four years with extreme highs and lows and endless unrealistic expectations of myself as a mother. I didn't need more control; I needed to gain back the woman who once loved openly and did not try to control her surroundings at all times. I had to make some changes, or I would go on living this uneasy bliss, never really having peace or feeling a sense of settled calm ever again. I was letting my past patterns and trauma dictate the kind of mother I had to be. I was an overwhelmed cluster of inward chaos who was putting on a smile.

If I was going to make a change, it would need to be the kind of change that takes place from the inside out. I am talking about grabbing a hold of myself and taking back my peace. The question was, did I truly want to stop my past patterns, heal my trauma, and have real peace, or was this just something to add to my task list to say I tried it? I had to commit, but the fear was taking over again. On the other hand, I really had nothing to lose and everything to gain because this chaotic clinging to control had to end.

The moment I decided to make change for myself was the moment my journey came full circle. I took the time to learn about what my soul needed. Mothering comes from the soul. We raise our children with our souls, not our lives. If we give them our whole lives, we ourselves will never have actually lived. I was mothering them from my head to protect my heart from fear and failure. I found out that the peace I was yearning for and this "control" that I thought I needed was actually easily found right at my fingertips. It was me needing to feed my soul daily.

Tip: Mindset work through positive affirmations, journaling, blessing and releasing people and thoughts that are not serving you, are all ways to ensure triggers lessen and patterns are not repeated.

Slowly, I began to break these patterns by replacing the rigidity of my routines with tasks that added to my growth as a mother. I went through guided meditations and constant prayer. I started journaling for three minutes a day, and I taught myself how to use positive affirmations effectively. I found myself again, and healing of past trauma has definitely taken place.

Am I perfect now? Gosh, no, and I may never be, but I am a better version of myself, healed from so many things I blamed myself for. People, circumstances, and events come into our lives for a season and a reason, and they leave for the same. Fear of not pleasing others and feeling vulnerable again was real for me -- fear of saying no to friends and family and fear of failure in my life, especially with my children. I was finally able to let go of all those past learned patterns.

If I have any other advice for anyone reading this, it is to stop and take your life back. Conquer the beasts that appear along your journey, and if you lose sight of who you are, stop and get her back. Always remember, it is our difficult journeys that teach us *real* purpose. Negative thoughts are naturally a place we visit, but if we learn not to set up camp and live in them, we can eventually live independently from them. Remember, you are meant for greatness. Don't let life's out of control events, unexpected twists and turns, and obstacles dim the light you are meant to shine.

My final words to whoever is reading my story are I am praying for you, and I pray you take some strength from my story when you feel you cannot go any farther. Know that you are loved, even when your heart is broken.

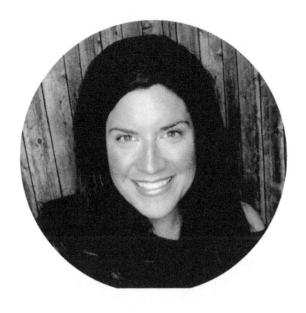

Scan the code for a video message from Cindy and a free gift

Cindy Grace is a mother of three children. She has twin 10-year-old sons and one 7-year-old daughter. Cindy's children are her true passion, and she loves spending her time ensuring that they are fulfilled. Cindy has a career as a speech-language pathologist but also deems herself an advocate for peaceful motherhood. Her infertility struggle began her motherhood journey, but due to her journey, advocacy for balance and peaceful mothering feeds her soul. During her 20 years as a speech-language pathologist, she has earned two master's degrees and a doctorate in a variety of areas of education.

To know Cindy is to know that she is loyal and loves her family and friends to her core. Cindy's hobby, turned side career, of helping peaceful driven moms find their balance is what has led her to write this chapter.

https://linktr.ee/cindygraceblog

INFERTILITY ALMOST WON

Kaila Stearns

Growing up, I always dreamed of becoming a mom. That dream only continued to grow as time dragged on. I often joked about using donor sperm, but all I really wanted was a family.

When my husband and I first started dating, I made a comment that started with, "When I have kids…". His response was, "You want kids?" You see, my husband already had a beautiful daughter who was 8, and he didn't want any more kids. My response to his question, of course, was, "Yes, do you?" Wouldn't you know, this man said, "I do now!"

It wasn't too long before we decided to start trying for a baby. You always hear of people getting pregnant right away or "it was only one time," so naturally, I assumed that it would happen that way for us, too. After a few months, I started using apps to track my cycle and ovulation. For a long time, I relied on the apps to tell me when I was ovulating. I researched about the female body and how our reproductive organs work. I used ovulation strips, which showed that I was ovulating differently than the apps said. I tried tracking my basal temp, even purchasing an internal basal thermometer that you put in every night before bed. I thought I was doing everything right, but why wasn't I pregnant?

I was so frustrated. I was finding myself more and more depressed every single month. I can't tell you how many times I would feel like it was finally **the** month and would take a pregnancy test … only for it to be negative. Inevitably, my period always seemed to show up the next day. There were other times when I just felt "different" at the time when I expected my period. I would take a pregnancy test, and there would be a faint line. I would take more tests, and there would still be a faint line, and then, my period would show her ugly face. They were always the worst periods, too. Crazy bad cramps, super heavy, and I felt like they would last a lifetime. After speaking with a doctor, I learned I was having chemical pregnancies. Eventually, I stopped taking tests, even if my period was a little late. I just couldn't take another let down.

TIP: If you think you might be experiencing chemical pregnancies, or know that you are, talk to your doctor to see if they can help pinpoint the cause. My doctors weren't able to find a cause. In the end, I found that mine were caused by having low blood sugar.

I had always had extremely heavy periods. Although, I didn't really know how heavy it was in comparison to a normal period. That's not something people really talk about. One day, I finally researched what a normal period looked like. Turns out, I was having a normal period's worth of bleeding within the first half hour of my period starting. I also had crazy painful cramps before, during, and sometimes in between my cycles. I would frequently have random pains that would drop me to my knees, and I would have to find a comfy position and stay there, or it would get worse. Growing up,

I went to countless doctors for all of the random symptoms I was having. I went to the same doctors multiple times as my symptoms would just continue to disrupt my life. I was always told that I was fine. It made me feel like I was crazy.

When I was 29 years old, I was being treated by a doctor for a migraine that I had been suffering from for 2 weeks straight, and my mom asked if he thought I could have endometriosis. We had been talking about other symptoms I was having with the migraine and just in general. I looked at her and said, "A what?" She went on to tell me that she had it when I was very young. She didn't suffer much before it was found and never had issues again after it was ablated, so she hadn't even thought about me having it.

After my mom mentioned endometriosis, I started researching, and I was convinced that it was, indeed, my problem. I went to see my new family doctor for a checkup, as my normal doctor had left the practice. When I met my new doctor, she was asking a ton of questions. I brought up endometriosis and our infertility. We had been trying to conceive for almost 2 years at this point. Since it had been over a year, she showed concern. She decided she would do an internal ultrasound to see if she could see anything. Why had nobody else ever thought to do this? She found that I have an arcuate uterus. Concerned, she sent me to a specialist.

The first visit with the specialist went great! She listened to me, didn't make me feel crazy, and she even decided that we needed to do an exploratory surgery to figure out what was going on. Upon completion of my exam, she said that she thought I had endometriosis. She sent us over to scheduling. For the first time in my life, I felt like I was finally going to get the help I needed. Three weeks later, I had surgery. I was so worried during the time leading up to the surgery that they would get in there and not find anything.

During my surgery, they found that I had stage 3 endometriosis. They removed a cyst from my left ovary, and they removed a bunch of adhesions that were webbed through the inside of my uterus. They didn't seem too worried about my arcuate uterus at that time, unless it posed problems in the future. The doctor said that she no longer saw anything stopping us from getting pregnant and recommended we start fertility treatments right away, so we did. We had three rounds of clomid and two failed IUIs. Before we knew the second one had failed, I went to the doctor to be seen as I felt like my ovaries were ginormous ... and they were. I was told that I had hyper stimulated ovaries. I had two different doctors tell me that when this happens, it generally means that the IUI worked. I left that doctor's office with my hopes soaring so high in the sky.

It hadn't meant that it worked ... shortly after that, mother nature decided to make her monthly visit. I was devastated. I was angry ... I was so angry. I found myself drowning my sorrows with alcohol. In fact, only days after our second failed IUI, I got really drunk and belligerent and made a complete fool of myself. It was then that I started getting my rear back to church and trying to get my life right.

Six months after the surgery that diagnosed my endometriosis, I was in a bad way all over again. I had my heating pad on all day and night, and I didn't have energy to do anything around the house; if I wasn't working, you could pretty much find me in bed. **Two months** later, I had another laparoscopy to remove the endometriosis that had grown or grown back. This time was with a different doctor. Before my surgery, he said, "Well, we will see." He wasn't fully convinced that my endometriosis had returned as aggressively as I was saying it had. At that moment, I felt much less confident in my decision to have another surgery. We went for it, though, and this time, I had stage 4 endometriosis that had infiltrated many more areas. It included my bladder, bowels, and rectum. When I woke up from surgery, I felt amazing, despite having just had surgery. I could just feel that it was all gone. There was one other problem; while he was in there, he found a hernia. Six weeks later, I had another surgery to repair the hernia.

Little did I know, five months later, I would be having yet another surgery. After having had four surgeries in only fourteen months, I decided it was time to take a break from trying to get pregnant. I just needed a break to heal. Infertility is so taxing; add the health issues, and I just couldn't take much more.

I started doing some new things to see if I could stay healthier longer. I was using essential oils and trying to rid my life of toxins. I was drinking a juice daily that was full of antioxidants, and I was eating a version of keto and paleo. I felt like I was on top of the world. I was cleaning my house and even did some painting. By the time we made it another seven or eight months, my symptoms had returned, and I was ready for another surgery.

This time, things were different. I didn't want to live my life having surgeries every six to eight months. After my first surgery up until this point, I did a lot of research. Many women had had success when they went to the endometriosis clinic in Georgia. I mean, why wouldn't they? These doctors have dedicated their lives to fighting endometriosis specifically. I decided to check them out. I filled out their crazy long application and was accepted. While I was going through the process of filling out the application and waiting to hear back from them, I just kept thinking about all the women who had hysterectomies, and it changed their lives.

I found myself doing even more research. I looked into the number of people helped by having hysterectomies vs. how many people the hysterectomies didn't change a thing or even made things worse. I know a couple people personally who have had hysterectomies because of endometriosis, and their lives were changed for the better, and they were so thankful they did it. I prayed and asked God for a sign, to show me the way. At this point, I was in a full-on battle with myself. Should I have another surgery to remove the endometriosis (and hopefully, finally get my quality of life back) and have the chance to become a mom. Or have a hysterectomy, which may make things better ... or worse ... and worst of all, lose my chance at ever having my little miracle baby/babies -- my biggest dream of all time! I reached out to the two people I knew who had hysterectomies to hear their stories and hopefully help me figure out what I was being called to do. I had asked God for a sign, and after chatting with them, I felt like I had my sign.

I decided to have a hysterectomy ...

I planned to call and schedule surgery that day. An hour after making the hardest decision I have ever made in my life, my mom called me. She tells me about how she went to this health store, and a guy there knew so much about endometriosis. My mom told me that I needed to talk to him right away. I became very upset. How dare she call me and throw something else into the mix when I had already made my decision. I called the man the next day and listened to what he had to say, but I did not buy it. The doctors didn't know enough about endometriosis to help me; how on earth could this guy help? He told me about a diet and testing that would tell me about my body chemistry.

The testing uses your saliva and urine to tell what your chemistry is. I decided to go to the store to have the testing done because, at this point, I really didn't have anything left to lose. I listened to the man as he told me things I had wrong with me that nobody else could have known. For instance, I didn't go around telling people that I suffered from confusion, yet this man somehow knew. Even crazier yet, he said, "You may not know this, but your body is conceiving and then kicking it right back out" (this is also known as a chemical pregnancy). Say what?! I decided I would try out this new diet/ lifestyle.

Within weeks of making recommended dietary and lifestyle changes, I was without pain, and I had much more energy. I was even able to deep clean my house. I would start to get ready for bed, and next thing I knew, I would find myself reorganizing a closet. Within two months, I was pregnant! We were over the moon! The pregnancy test line was the darkest it has ever been. We even made it past the 5-week mark which was the furthest along we had ever been. That pregnancy did end in miscarriage. Something strange happened, though. Normally, this miscarriage would have turned me upside down for some time. But I took a day to grieve, and that following day, I got up, and I decided that I wasn't going to let my grief take over. I started cleaning the house and went about my day as if it were any other day. I even went to a festival that weekend to look at all the pretty tulips that are grown in a small town in Iowa.

I had given everything to God in a way that I never had before. In the past, I would lay things at his feet and then pick them right back up. This time, I didn't pick it back up. I had a new found hope ... unwavering faith.

The following month, we were pregnant **again**!

If I said I didn't have moments of fear, I would be lying. When I found myself in those moments of worry, I would remind myself that God is in control, not me. I can't tell you how many times in a day I would say to him, "Your will be done."

My pregnancy was not smooth sailing as I had always imagined it would be. From the day I found out I was pregnant until about 16 weeks, I was having issues with low blood sugar. Thankfully, at this point, I already knew it was something I needed to keep a close eye on. I experienced spotting starting at 5 weeks along and bled heavily multiple times before we reached 12 weeks. Were those times scary? Absolutely! In each moment, I was terrified … each time I found myself there, I would pray the same prayer and just trust that God had everything under control.

We ran into some other things along the way that caused some fear to resurface. I just kept praying that same prayer and trusting that God would bring our baby boy to us happy and healthy. Knowing, believing … fully trusting that God would do these things is what got me through!

I thought for sure this very strong-willed little boy that was growing inside of me would make his debut early! I should have known better … he came after his due date. And not without a fight.

On an evening in February, six years after we started trying … we brought our beautiful baby boy, Bradley, into the world.

Never give up hope! I found that when I truly surrendered, that's when things really started falling into place.

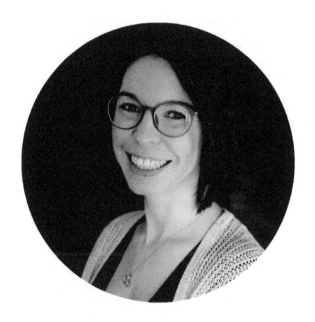

Scan the code for a video message from Kaila and a free gift

Kaila Stearns is a business strategist, executive assistant, fertility coach, wife and blessed mama.

She currently resides in Iowa with her husband, bonus daughter, son, and their six animals (4 dogs and 2 cats). She is passionate about serving women who are struggling with infertility, especially those who also have endometriosis, to help them heal and overcome their hurdles.

Kaila spent almost six years of her life researching ... trying all the diets, trends, and treatments in an effort to achieve fertility. She can't wait to help you avoid some of those steps and looks forward to watching you kick infertility to the curb.

kailastearns.com/links

THE FAMILY WE WERE MEANT TO BE

Laura Watson

L ooking back, I always assumed children were in my future, but I was almost forty-one years old when my husband, Jared, and I were married and ready to start a family. At the recommendation of my primary care doctor, I visited an obstetrician for blood work to get an idea of what issues we might face while trying to conceive. I went to that appointment excited to get started on building a family, but even before the results were available, she looked at me and said, "I don't know how important this is to you, but I don't see many women over 40 who get pregnant with their own eggs." Her words stung, but the visit forced me to examine how strongly I wanted children and what avenues we were willing to explore in order to start a family.

The results of the blood work showed that this was, indeed, going to be difficult. My AMH (or anti-müllerian hormone) level was very low, even lower than expected for a woman my age. Since this hormone reflects a woman's ovarian reserve or quantity of eggs, it was recommended I seek treatment from a reproductive endocrinologist right away, so we dove into the world of reproductive medicine.

TIP: Be open to all the options and discuss them with your partner.

I'm thankful that my husband and I decided early on to consider all options and not dismiss any possibilities without a discussion. In the beginning, it was hard to imagine anything beyond the traditional methods of family building, but knowing that we were both open to alternatives gave me hope and helped me move forward when treatments didn't work. Having an open dialogue together ultimately led us to finding the best path to complete our family.

I spent the next year trying all the treatments, reading all the literature, learning all the acronyms, and battling lots of disappointment when therapies and procedures were unsuccessful. We tried a few medicated cycles with the oral drug, Clomid, with no success but a lot of headaches due to the increased hormones. We then moved to an IUI cycle, which was also unsuccessful. Months had come and gone, and we were no closer to having a baby. I had hoped that maybe one of these less invasive therapies would work, but when a second attempt at an IUI resulted in a negative pregnancy test, our doctor was ready to get us started on our first IVF cycle.

It was both exciting and daunting to start IVF. At first, I thought for sure that we would soon be pregnant. I even looked through a calendar and tried to predict when a baby might be due. Little did I know it would be months before we would even start a cycle.

The day my stimulation medications arrived, I opened the box like it was a much-anticipated gift on Christmas morning, hoping the vials and syringes would be the key to success. My clinic offered a session to carefully go through my instructions, but I was still intimidated on the first night I had to give myself an injection. Online, I found forums, blog posts, and YouTube videos with advice on how to properly give myself the meds and manage any side effects like headaches, nausea, or irritability. I was determined to be a perfect patient and follow my protocol as closely as possible because it was one of the only things, I had control over.

> *Tip: Look for resources to help guide you with the medications. When I starting an IVF protocol, the medication instructions can be overwhelming. I would advise someone starting treatment to request time with a nurse at the clinic or another trusted resource to go over how to properly prepare and administer the medications. If you have a partner, have them get comfortable with the medications, so they can help with some of the trickier injections. Some of the medications can be unpleasant, but they are important for a successful cycle. Trust that you can do it and believe that it will all be worth it.*

Our hopes were high for our first attempt at an egg retrieval, and I was optimistic that it would lead to a baby. The procedure resulted in only three eggs, but I wasn't discouraged. "It only takes one," I told myself.

The next day, when a nurse called to let us know that all three eggs had been fertilized, I jumped for joy but sadly only one embryo made it to day 5. For a week, we waited while our one embryo was sent for preimplantation genetic testing (PGT) and hoped we would soon be preparing for an embryo transfer. Instead, our doctor called to share that the embryo tested positive for a chromosome abnormality and would not result in a viable pregnancy. Even though I tried to prepare myself for this scenario, it was crushing to hear. I didn't give myself time to grieve the failure of the cycle, I just wanted to try again.

Our doctor made very few changes to my protocol, and I had hoped that after some experience, this cycle would go a little better, but that was not the case. The second egg retrieval resulted in just two eggs, neither of which survived long enough to possibly be transferred.

On the way to the clinic for my third egg retrieval, I shook my head and said, "This is never going to work." It was uncharacteristic of me to be so negative, and Jared was surprised by my attitude, but something inside me knew that we were spinning our wheels. My prediction was correct. Just like the prior two procedures, the egg retrieval failed to produce an embryo that would someday be a baby.

We were now a year into our infertility journey, and I was another year older. I was frustrated and discouraged that every treatment we had tried so far was a failure. Another doctor we met shared that given my extremely low egg count, he believed I had the same chances at a successful pregnancy on my own as with IVF. Either way, those chances were very unlikely. He did not recommend we continue IVF treatment, at least not with my own eggs. Leaving the office, Jared asked me if I was okay after receiving such a difficult message. I smiled at him and said that I was fine. Honestly, I was much better than fine. We were about to turn a corner on our journey to becoming parents.

Tip: Trust your instincts. I knew after three unsuccessful egg retrievals that we needed to move in a new direction. I felt very fortunate that my instincts to move to donor egg IVF were so strong. There is such an abundance of information available that it can become overwhelming and confusing for someone who is unsure about the right decision for their family. I would advise anyone in this position to surround themselves with medical professionals that support their goals and also to trust what their heart tells them.

I had already begun researching donor egg IVF, and, after getting used to the idea, it sparked new hope. It was hard to come to terms with having a baby that would have another woman's genetics instead of mine, but Jared said something that helped me let that go. He reminded me my strongest traits, such as kindness, empathy, and patience, would be passed on with nurturing and parenting, not DNA.

It didn't take me long to find the right donor, based on photos and a detailed questionnaire. We chose a young woman who had physical characteristics similar to mine, like fair skin and blue eyes. More importantly, her questionnaire answers were sensitive and sincere, focused on her love for family and a passion for helping people.

Working with our IVF clinic, a donor agency, and contract attorneys, we were soon off and running. For the first time in a long while, I was filled with hope. I sat in our doctor's office and said with absolute certainty, "This is going to work. This is how we are going to get our family."

Over the next few months, I sat on the sidelines, trusting an anonymous woman I didn't know to take over crucial steps in conceiving our child. After each of her monitoring appointments, the nurse would call me to share how she was responding. Initially, I feared the positive updates might make me resentful or jealous, but with every call, I became more thankful and appreciative of what she was doing for us. I wished I could thank her myself but instead asked our nurse to share my gratitude.

The donor's egg retrieval was a success. Five days later, my doctor transferred one perfect embryo. After having gone through 18 months of disappointment and heartbreak, I finally experienced my first positive pregnancy test. While it would be poetic to say, "I couldn't believe it," it was no surprise. I knew this would work with a feeling just as strong as I'd felt months before.

The following August our son, Duke, was born. He looks remarkably like Jared and is impressively coordinated for a child his age, so we are confident he has Daddy's athletic ability. Like me, he loves books, music, and has a giggle that is no doubt a parrot of mine. He is, without question, my son.

Our story and struggle didn't end there. When Duke was just 9 months old, I suffered a miscarriage. In an ironic twist of fate, I had become pregnant on my own. I hadn't even realized something was off since my cycles were still irregular. One morning, I believed that I had started my period, but it rapidly became clear that something was very wrong. I stared in disbelief at a positive pregnancy test but knew I was experiencing a loss. An ultrasound showed no evidence of life. My feelings regarding this loss were complex and still are years later. I felt guilty that a baby was trying to grow inside me, and I didn't even know he or she was there.

While coming to terms with the loss, we decided we were ready for another baby to complete our family. We saw our doctor and put together a plan to transfer one of the frozen embryos we were fortunate to have from our donor cycle. I felt incredibly optimistic after the transfer and wasn't surprised at all when I had a positive pregnancy test a week later.

The early symptoms of pregnancy began to arrive, and I was giddy with anticipation for a new baby. At seven weeks, Jared and I arrived at our clinic, excited for the early ultrasound, but the doctor had some concerns. They struggled to find a consistent heart rate, and the readings were low. We were told to come back for a follow-up the next week.

Seven days later, I was hopeful for better results, but what we learned was shocking. There were two heartbeats! The transferred embryo had split, and I was carrying identical twins. Relief that I was still pregnant was quickly replaced with concern over carrying twins and having three babies under two. We were terrified but slowly adjusting to the idea of becoming a family of five when we went back to the clinic for an ultrasound just shy of 10 weeks.

It was then that the emotional roller coaster we had been on came to a screeching halt as the sonographer said to us, "I'm sorry, but I don't see a viable pregnancy." The babies were gone. Further testing revealed that they were positive for trisomy 13, an abnormality that we would have found ahead of time had we elected for PGT testing. However, since our donor was young and healthy, it seemed like an unnecessary risk to our embryos and expense, but I began to wonder if it was a mistake.

It was devastating to lose this pregnancy. It was just a couple of weeks before Christmas, and I had planned to announce our news to our families with a letter from Santa to Duke, congratulating him on having such a wonderful year and then "promoting" him to Big Brother. Inside, I was sad all the time and battling physical discomfort like the migraine headaches caused by a sudden drop in hormone levels, but it was the holidays. We were visiting family, and I had a toddler who needed me, so I did everything I could to put on a brave face and keep my pain to myself.

All I wanted to do was move forward, but we took a short break after the loss to allow my body to heal as well as my broken heart. When we were ready to try again, the world began to shut down due to the Covid-19 pandemic. We were able to transfer another embryo that spring, but it resulted in a negative pregnancy test, likely due to another abnormal embryo. A third frozen embryo transfer resulted in yet another loss very early in my pregnancy.

I asked my doctor if we made a mistake in not testing the embryos and if we should test them now. He understood that I was becoming frustrated and nervous that we would never have another baby, but he also believed testing now would be risky to our embryos. I knew he was right, and we kept going.

In the fall of 2020, a fourth frozen embryo transfer resulted in a positive pregnancy test. I was happy but frightened. The losses had taken a toll on me, and I developed anxiety, which I learned was very common for women who are pregnant after loss. I was terrified of losing another baby and struggled to focus on anything beyond my fear. Once again, I kept my feelings to myself and saved tears for times when I was alone, determined not to burden anyone with my emotions.

Then, as I began the second trimester, I realized I wasn't allowing myself to enjoy the pregnancy I had wanted so badly. I was putting worry ahead of my joy. The baby I was carrying deserved better and so did I. My doctor assured me that my feelings were valid and normal. She also applauded me for communicating my needs. Her office helped me schedule some time with a staff social worker and planned my office visits no further than three weeks apart, so I never had to go long without hearing a heartbeat. I also started a prenatal safe fitness routine, including daily yoga to feel physically healthy and strong. Eventually, I began to feel movement on a regular basis, and while my anxiety never fully went away, the little kicks told me that a healthy baby was growing inside me.

The first time I saw my daughter, I knew this was the way it was meant to be. I will always mourn my losses, but this little girl was the baby I was meant to hold in my arms.

> *TIP: The anxiety that comes along with pregnancy after loss is complicated, and the emotions are conflicting. When I began to open up about my anxiety and actively seek out tools and support to help me manage it, I was able to start enjoying that special time preparing for our daughter rather than worrying that I would never meet her. Part of my hesitation in talking about my feelings was that I was supposed to be happy. After three difficult losses, I was finally going to have a baby. However, it's not that easy, and I had to allow myself to feel everything -- the sadness for my losses, the fear that nothing was guaranteed, and the excitement for the baby I was carrying. I would advise any family in this position to proactively discuss their feelings and be open about any fears. There is no shame in examining your feelings and talking through emotions, especially if it could benefit your emotional health at such a vulnerable time.*

We have already begun sharing Duke's story with him and will do the same with our daughter, Quinn. We keep it simple for a young mind and focus on how much we appreciate everyone who helped us bring them here. We thank the doctors, the nurses, and, particularly, the special woman who gave us the very important eggs that helped to make them before they grew inside mommy. We talk about how it took three of us, daddy, mommy, and our very generous donor, to create our family, and we are so grateful that it turned out the way it did.

As our children grow and mature, we will offer more details and answer all questions, so they are aware of how they came to be and why it's special. It is our goal that they never find our story strange or shameful, and if they become curious about the anonymous woman with whom they share DNA, we will tell them what we know and navigate the inquiries truthfully.

For five years, much of my life revolved around pregnancy -- trying to get pregnant, wishing I was pregnant, and being pregnant. The journey was long, challenging, and both emotionally and physically difficult. I'm not sure I knew how mentally strong I was before our pursuit to start a family, but looking back, I'm so thankful I was able to move ahead after each setback. I knew I was meant to bring these children into the world and stopped at nothing to make that happen. Now that they are here, they are more perfect than I could have ever dreamed. I can't imagine any other outcome, and I wouldn't change a thing.

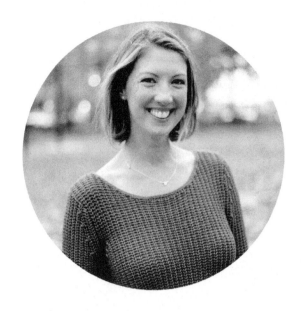

Scan the code for a video message from Laura and a free gift

Laura Watson is a freelance writer, storyteller, and avid reader. From a young age, she has always enjoyed the art of words on a page. She found ways to incorporate her talent into a professional career with non-profit organizations and sharing her experience as a distance runner and triathlete on a personal blog. Today, Laura's work is focused on relationships, motherhood, the challenge of raising compassionate children in our modern world, her experience with infertility treatments and pregnancy loss. A native of New England, she loves the change of seasons, traveling, fitness, and books of all kinds. She lives in Boston with her husband, Jared, and two beautiful children.

https://linktr.ee/laura.watson

DRAGONFLY DREAMS AND LITTLE BOY KISSES

Saskia Williams

My infertility journey started back when I was just 27 years old. I never wanted to be an old mom, and so, after six months of marriage, we started trying to conceive.

After six months, being the controlling type of person that I am (I'm sure most women going through this journey can relate), I took myself off to my GP. We were living in the UK at the time, and our male GP told me that we needed to try for at least 12 months before coming back for a referral to a fertility clinic. That wasn't good enough for me (surprise surprise), so I made an appointment with a female GP and got our referral to the closest fertility clinic.

Tip: Always follow your gut instincts; you know your body best. Push for the care you deserve, and find someone who listens to your concerns.

After a few tests on me and a sperm test, we were diagnosed as having male infertility and referred for ICSI. Once they diagnosed David, they ceased their testing on me. Interestingly, now that I know as much as I do, I know that should not have happened; all tests should be carried out on both parties, so the full picture is available. A few (wasted) years later, I was diagnosed as having a low ovarian reserve. That could have been picked up earlier had I had the full realm of tests.

In the seven years, we had only three IVF treatments. We were naïve during our first cycle; we were so sure that it would work that we weren't emotionally prepared at all to deal with a negative outcome.

The negative pregnancy test that came along with that cycle really shocked us, and we had a long talk afterwards about our expectations going forwards. We decided that we would only do three cycles in total, not just due to financial reasons but also due to emotional ones. We said we would throw everything we could at the cycles, we would do everything right, and if by the third, nothing happened, we would get off the crazy train. All specialists generally say to allow for at least three cycles, and that's why, over the seven years, we only completed three cycles of IVF.

> *Tip: Only you know what your limit is. I have known people who have drawn a line at one cycle and others who have done 15+, but it is good to keep the lines of communication open and to be on the same page with your partner.*

We flew to South Africa for our next treatment, two years after our first cycle failed. This time, we had two embryos make it to day 5, and we left the clinic and the country with the specialist's words ringing in our ears," Prepare yourself for twins." So, two weeks later, when we got our second negative test result, we both fell apart emotionally.

In 2009, my sister had a baby girl. They got married a few years after us and decided to start trying to get pregnant earlier than they had planned to because of the struggles we were having. Within three months, they were pregnant, but I will never forget how they told us they were pregnant. We got a call from my parents, who were having a braai (BBQ) with my sister and brother-in-law. After a chat, my mom handed the phone over to my sister, telling me that she had something to tell me. Instinctively, I knew ... and I didn't react well. I tried to keep them from hearing the tears in my voice, but I couldn't, and after congratulating her, I handed the phone over to David.

I couldn't stop thinking, why couldn't my sister call me privately or message me at least? Why do it in "public" out of the blue? Later that week, my mother called me selfish and told me that I had upset my sister. No one even thought about how I felt. I didn't speak to my sister her entire pregnancy, and I actually don't think I have ever truly forgiven her for that.

Tip: No one is going to understand how it feels to be infertile, unless they have been through it. Try to find a support group of women or men going through the journey. I had an online forum that helped me through my final cycle and through everything that followed.

In 2010, we made the decision to apply to adopt. Adoption was never a last resort for us. We planned to have one biological child and then complete our family through adoption. We all know how best laid plans go, don't we?

At the same, we decided to move to South Africa (I am South African, and David is British), and so we started the adoption there in 2011. The process is invasive, but you can get onto the list within six weeks if you do all the paperwork in a timely fashion, and we got onto the adoption list in November 2011.

Once we had something in place should our final IVF fail, I was then ready for our third and final IVF cycle and began the process in May 2012. Prior to starting the cycle, I went to see a medium. I know many people don't believe in them or tarot cards, etc., but I needed to try and get answers in any way that I could. Infertility treatment makes you totally obsessive and desperate to try and regain even a sliver of control. My gran had died the year before, and she had known what we were going through, but she was a very strict Catholic and would never even have entertained the idea of a medium. However, my gran also knew how much I needed to know what she had to tell me, and she came through and told me that we would have a baby boy by the end of the year. Considering it was May, even if we had gotten pregnant by June/July when our cycle ended, we wouldn't have the baby by the end of the year, but I didn't dwell on that. I focused on the fact that we were going to have a baby!!

I also joined an online support group that had monthly cycle buddy rooms, which really helped me in the lead up cycle and what came afterwards. Back in the UK, I was also part of an online forum. The girls supported without judging, and as I knew no one else going through infertility at the time, it really was a lifeline.

As it was our final try, we used donor sperm, as well as my husband's, and we did a ZIFT procedure, which is pretty invasive but is proven to work well in cases of male infertility.

The cycle ended in my first ever pregnancy! This is it, we thought, we have done it!

Then came our first hurdle … the beta levels didn't rise as expected. Our specialist recommended no more beta tests and to rather do an early scan. The scan was fine; there was a sac in the correct place (so not an ectopic), but it was too early for a heartbeat.

Then came our week 7 scan, where we were super excited to hear our baby's heartbeat. However, the sac had collapsed, and the specialist told us it was more than likely a miscarriage but to come in for weekly scans free of charge, so we could monitor the situation. Miraculously, our baby caught up and was perfect by our 12-week anatomy scan.

We had a gender reveal party just after our 17-week scan, which still ranks as one of the best days of my life. Our family took turns guessing what sex the baby would be, and my husband and I were so sure we were having a boy after what my gran had said through the medium that we nearly fell over backwards when the cake revealed pink icing. We then spent the following day excitedly going through potential girls' names and we chose Eloise. A beautiful name for our beautiful girl. It was at the 20-week scan that our world came crashing down. There was something wrong with our little girl's brain. Thinking back, our OB/GYN definitely picked something up at our 17-week scan, but as we had revealed our plans for the gender reveal party, he let us have our few weeks of joy before the pain he knew was coming. We will always be grateful to him for that. Her ventricles were swollen twice as much as the normal range for girls. Our fetal assessment scan was moved up to the next day. There, we found out that the enlargements could be due to a blockage, which would be cured by a shunt, as everything else was growing normally. We did an amniocentesis to rule out any chromosomal abnormalities, but the specialist was relatively positive about the outcome, and we started to breathe again.

On the 15th November, 2012, at 8 a.m., the fetal specialist called us and told us that our daughter had a chromosomal abnormality not compatible with life.

After crying buckets full of tears, we decided to consult with the geneticist who did the tests, as she would be able to clarify the situation better. She explained that neither myself nor my husband are carriers of translocated chromosomes and that Eloise's unbalanced configuration (i.e.: 2, 7, and 20) is extremely rare, and, without us being carriers, the chances of our daughter getting it were 1 in a million!! Once again, we were at the bad end of a statistic. Without the enlarged ventricles (hydrocephalus), the chances of severe birth defects would be 50%, but with the hydrocephalus, they became over 80%.

> *Tip: PGD testing on embryos was very new in South Africa at that time, and as neither of us had any issues, we didn't think of doing it, but now, I recommend it to everyone.*

We booked an MRI to get a better picture of her brain and idea of possible damage. We also went for a 3D scan to spend time with our brave daughter who had already defied the odds, and we knew if anyone could turn this around, she could. We were not giving up on her.

The results of the MRI weren't good news. The ventricles were now 65% bigger than normal range just a few weeks on from our fetal assessment, and we still had 16 weeks left of the pregnancy. The prognosis was very bad.

Determined, we consulted with the head of genetics at WITS and phoned a professor in the USA who was touted to be the top geneticist in the world. They all came back with the same prognosis. All the specialists agreed that it would be cruel to bring her into this world to suffer a short life, full of pain. We had hit a brick wall.

Terminating for medical reasons was not a term I was familiar with until we came face to face with the decision that no parent should ever have to make. We went to see our OB/GYN and sat with him for an hour, discussing everything and making the final decision together.

He organized the termination for late the next day, when the hospital would be quieter, and he put together a special team as, understandably, not all medical staff want to be involved in such a harrowing operation. I told him I wanted to give birth to her naturally, but he explained as gently as he could that it may damage her swollen head, and then, we wouldn't be able to see her or to take pictures of her. He sent us home to spend the next 20 hours with our baby girl.

The 22nd November, 2012, dawned as a rainy day. We danced with our girl in the rain, we listened to and recorded her heartbeat, we read to her, we took family pictures, and we officially named her Eloise Iris Seanna Williams. Iris is a name on both sides of the family, and Seanna means "God has given."

Mothers of babies who didn't make it into our arms are huge carriers of guilt. What could I have done differently? It has to be my fault; it happened in my belly! Now, just imagine the guilt of a mother who has to make the decision to end her daughter's life. As long as I live, I will never, ever get over having to do that.

In the days following her death, we saw signs from her; more specifically, we saw dragonflies, which we had never really seen as we don't live near water. They appeared in our garden, flying next to our cars while we drove, and anywhere we visited. When we looked up the meaning of seeing so many dragonflies, we found that a dragonfly represents" a short life well lived," and they tend to appear to many people after a loved one dies. People have believed for many generations that it's a sign that your loved one is okay where their soul now resides. We took it as a sign of forgiveness and love from our Eloise, and it soothed our shattered souls a bit.

I was signed off from work for the rest of the year to heal from my operation, as well as work through all my emotions.

I phoned our social worker, Zoe, to let her know what had happened as she holds back adoption profiles from biological parents when the adopter is pregnant and until the parents are ready to adopt as an option for their second child (like we had always planned). When she first told us that they pause their search until you have a live birth, I was confused in my naivety … Now I know exactly why they do it; after all, 1 in 4 pregnancies end in a loss.

Three weeks after Eloise died, I was at home alone, just going through the motions, completely cocooned in my own grief. It was around 4 p.m. in the afternoon when my phone rang, and Zoe's name flashed up. Zoe was the most amazing human being. I was sure she was just calling to check up on me and to see how we were doing, but after she asked after us both, she told me that there was a baby whose biological mother had chosen our profile as first choice. I was floored with a mix of emotions. When you are on the adoption list, you imagine how THE CALL will go, the one when your social worker phones you and tells you about *your baby's* existence. In your imagination, it's always an immensely happy phone call, with shrieks of joy and excitement, but you never imagine that the call would come just 3 weeks after the most traumatic loss of your entire life. I could hardly process what she was saying.

The baby was a boy; Zoe said she would never have put us forward for a girl, as she knew that would be too much for us to cope with. She very nearly didn't put our profile in, as it was so soon after Eloise went to heaven, but as there were 13 other eligible profiles being sent, she knew the chances were slim that we would be picked, so she sent it in and left it in God's hands. I was silent throughout this exchange, so she continued on with the information that there was a second and third choice too, so if we felt it was too soon, we shouldn't worry that the little boy would be homeless. She told me to speak to David when he got home and to call her in the morning. I called David straight away and asked him where he was … He was 5 minutes away. After the longest 5 minutes of my life, he walked in, and we just fell into each other's arms and cried and cried. When we pulled ourselves together, I explained what Zoe had said and that she said it was completely our decision whether or not it was too soon to bring a baby into our home.

We talked most of the night, and we decided that this little boy was a gift, not from God but from Eloise. Their souls would have crossed paths in heaven, and she sent him down to be with her mommy and daddy, as she couldn't.

We called Zoe in the morning, and we made a time to meet with her that day, to hear the background and information about the baby boy, and to talk to her before making our final decision.

During that talk and after hearing all about him, David and I made our mutual decision by squeezing each other's hands under the table, and we told Zoe that we would be his parents.

We decided that we needed to start therapy as soon as possible as parenting a newborn whilst dealing with the kind of grief we were dealing with, both the loss of Eloise and the guilt over the decision we made, would be difficult. We owed it to this little soul to work on ourselves to be the best parents to him that we could be.

Ashton came home three days later, when he was just 10 days old. Our son is now a bright, handsome and bubbly 9-year-old. He knows his story, Zoe was very clear that it needed to be a part of his narrative from the beginning, so it's just normal for him. Our family and friends adore him, and we obviously adore him, too.

He is sociable and makes friends easily. He has been diagnosed as intellectually gifted, and we couldn't be prouder of him.

What I learned during our journey, and through the years that have followed, is that there are many paths to parenthood when you are infertile … the general ones: IUI, IVF, and ICSI, and the next level ones: egg/sperm donation, surrogacy, and adoption. During some of them, you may lose the chance for your child to have your genes, but all of them have the same end goal, to make you a family.

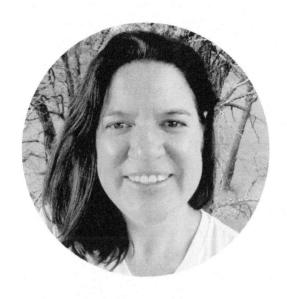

Scan the code for a video message from Saskia and a free gift

During 2013, a group of 10 infertile women started a nonprofit organization called The Infertility Awareness Association of South Africa, the first infertility charity of its kind in South Africa. Saskia co-founded it, in Eloise's memory, to make her proud of her mommy.

IFAASA advocates for fair coverage from our South African Medical Insurance as treatment for infertility is excluded on most of them. They educate the public through events, seminars and campaigns to break the stigma surrounding infertility.

Now, Saskia is the last active founding member and director. One by one, the others left to spend time with their miracle babies. There are days when Saskia thinks about doing the same, because working a full-time job, as well as running an NPO, is hard, but after experiencing what she did to get to her family of 4, she can't give up on helping others

During the past year, IFAASA has won a fight against South Africa's biggest medical aid, and after numerous meetings in 2020, they included coverage for treatment on some plans, starting January 2021. They have also been chosen to be founding members of the World Fertility Organization, launching in 2022.

This is Saskia's purpose and passion; please contact her if there is anything she can do to help you through your journey.

https://linktr.ee/ifaasa

https://linktr.ee/fertilitycoachsouthafrica

LOSING HOPE AND FINDING FAITH

Amanda Ignot

As a young woman, I dreamed of being a mom. I even remember writing out unique names for my future kids, always a little different, of course.

At 14, I remember saying I didn't want to have kids after I turned 30. I didn't want to be the "old mom". I'm not really sure what I thought I knew back then, but one thing is certain: I wanted to be a mom someday. Though I realize now that I was a bit naive back then, I hadn't been too concerned about being a young mother.

When I was 20, I got married. Though we weren't trying to get pregnant right away, we weren't doing a good job of trying to prevent it either, and in November of that year, I found out I was expecting. It was admittedly a shock, but I excitedly shared the news with my family at our holiday gathering.

In late December, I started spotting. I went to the hospital to have blood work done, then had to go back again a few days later to have it repeated. The waiting, both in between and after the second blood draw, was horrible. I was a basket case, scared and anxious to know what was going on.

I wasn't experiencing cramping or any other signs of miscarriage, but I was scared. It seemed like it took forever for my doctor's office to call with the results. Ironically, as soon as I got the phone call that confirmed I was, in fact, losing my baby, I started cramping. The next few days were the hardest days of my life. On January 4, 1997, I lost my first child to a miscarriage.

While in the throes of my miscarriage, my young husband had no idea how to help, so he went to work. I suffered the loss alone. Our baby wasn't real for him yet, and honestly, he just didn't know how to be there for me.

The weeks that followed were hard. I tried to get back to living my life, but knowing that I wouldn't be welcoming a baby in July was heartbreaking and seeing pregnant women everywhere was more than I could handle. I cried myself to sleep every night for weeks, crying out all the questions that were haunting me and wishing my baby was safe in my womb still.

After the miscarriage, my husband asked me to go on birth control. We hadn't planned on getting pregnant and, having just faced that reality, he didn't feel like we were ready for that stage. I saw my doctor for the follow-up, and he said we could try to get pregnant again right away if I wanted, but I chose to go on the pill instead. I don't think I was ready, and I wanted to make sure I didn't suffer another loss like that again anytime soon.

By early 1999, I had separated from my husband and was single again, and in April of 2000, I stopped taking the pill. I had started dating and moved in with my boyfriend later that year. We were together for six years. We did nothing to prevent pregnancy, and since he had a daughter from a previous relationship, I knew he could get someone pregnant. But not me.

In 2006, I took a job in another state. He didn't want to move, so we ended our six-year relationship and I moved on. After that, I was at a point in my life that I wanted to be a mom, and quite frankly, I didn't care if I was in a relationship or not. There were a few relationships after that (one for a year and a half and another for 6 months), and I never took steps to prevent becoming pregnant. But still, no baby.

No positive pregnancy tests, no late periods, nothing at all!! I was frustrated. I began to think I would never be able to have children. My cycles were regular, and I had no health problems that I was aware of. **What was wrong with me?**

The one common denominator was me.

In late 2009, I met Jonathan. We started dating in December, and I knew this time was different. I was in my early 30s, ready to settle down, and was so happy that he wanted too as well. We decided to try for a baby and had all the fun that goes into getting pregnant (wink, wink). But again, **nothing** happened.

Things got rough between us. I lost my self-confidence over the months of not getting pregnant, and he was tired of waiting, thinking I wouldn't be able to give him children. He also missed who I was when we met. Everything in my life focused on getting pregnant and making him happy. He was (and is) the love of my life. I was scared of losing him. In 2011, I started seeking answers and was told that tracking my cycles was the first step in addressing whether there was a problem.

> *TIP: Use an app to track your cycle so that you can start the conversations with your OBGYN early on. This will help you be ahead of the game, since the more you know about your cycle, the faster you will be able to enlist the support of fertility help.*

The stress through each cycle, and the disappointment every time my period showed up, had me losing hope of ever having a child. I kept going, holding my breath again and again each month, because I desperately wanted to be a mother. I also wanted my relationship to work. I didn't want to end up alone, a woman never having a marriage that lasted, never realizing her dream of being a mom. If I couldn't conceive, my future looked solemn and gray, where I would be lonely with nobody to love me unconditionally.

Jonathan and I split briefly in the fall of 2011, but then were married on January 1, 2012. It might sound crazy, but I guess when you love something, you have to let it go and hope that it loves you enough to come back!

In December 2011, I started a new job, we got a new place together, and I was finally able to see a fertility specialist. Through our journey so far, we had determined that:

1. I do ovulate every month
2. things were okay with my husband

The next step was to determine if my tubes were blocked, so I was sent to get a hysterosalpingography (HSG.) Let me tell you a little something about that experience…

It was freezing cold in the x-ray room, I was shaking with emotions and nerves, and I bawled the entire time. It was painful when they inserted the catheter and injected the dye, and in the end, they were only able to get clear x-rays of one of my tubes.

> *TIP: If you have to do this procedure, take someone with you for emotional support! This is not a procedure you want to go through on your own.*

Thoughts that were running through my head that day included:

"What if my tubes are blocked?"

"Is this the end for me?"

"What will happen to our marriage?"

"Am I ever going to be a mom?"

If my tubes were blocked, then that would be the end of the fertility road for us. IVF was not an option; we couldn't afford it. I was terrified of the results, wished they would give feedback right then and there to ease my mind. The HSG results determined that at least one of my tubes was not blocked. I was so relieved! This meant there were still other options to explore before IVF would be recommended.

From here, I started taking three medications at specific times and orders throughout my cycles:

1. Clomid to increase FSH (follicle stimulating hormone) and LH production (luteinizing hormone),
2. Estradiol to support my natural estrogen levels, and
3. Prometrium to support progesterone levels after insemination.

Taking these medications was the start of our intrauterine insemination (IUI) journey. We decided to try just the meds for a month, followed by an IUI, and repeated that schedule for seven months. During this time, I underwent four IUI procedures.

NOTE: Most doctors will only perform an IUI three times, but because there was no underlying reason why I wasn't getting pregnant, my doctor attempted a fourth try at my request.

TIP: If your doctor offers IUI as an option for you, ask how many procedures they are willing to perform. Consider another doctor if they say less than three.

I went in for my fourth and final IUI (my last chance) two days before my 37th birthday. If you have ever been through this process or been trying to get pregnant, you know that the two week wait after IUI to determine success or failure is the hardest and longest part of the journey! I knew I needed to focus on what was in my control and not get anxious over what was or wasn't happening in my body. That said, I would be lying if I said I wasn't a nervous wreck!

I was exercising daily and had been steadily losing weight, feeling great, slimming down and toning up. I had even just bought a bunch of new clothes in smaller sizes in the weeks leading up to that final IUI. (In hindsight, I guess it's kind of like washing your car right before it rains!)

There was a rift between us and it felt like we were worlds apart. I was working out to prove something, to feel better about myself, and to keep my mind off of what we were walking through. There was a lack of communication and connection emotionally and I felt like I was going through this whole process alone. Honestly, looking back,

I wouldn't have been surprised if he walked out. He made me feel like our home was the last place he wanted to be.

The two-week wait was over! Day 1 of my cycle came and went with no period. Day after day, I waited. Finally, I messaged my doctor and let her know that I hadn't gotten my period but that I was too scared to test. She told me to just go ahead and test; she couldn't understand why I was hesitant and nervous.

I was afraid that it was just wishful thinking and that the test would be negative again or, even worse, that as soon as I tested, my period would start. I'm sure I'm not the only one that has felt this way through this process, right?

Four days later, I went home and did my usual workout, followed by a walk on the treadmill. I noticed that I had to stop walking for a second time to use the restroom. I decided to go ahead and take a test.

I wanted to vomit during the whole 5-minute wait! I paced around our tiny apartment, trying to control my anxiety as my test strip processed, trying so hard not to go look before it was time.

It was the longest and most difficult 5 minutes of my life, and finally, it was time to look. Have you ever crept up on a test strip, trying to look and not look at the same time? That was me in that moment, and I bet I looked pretty ridiculous had anyone been watching!

The test was positive! I hit the floor and praised GOD, in Spanish, no less (which is not even my first language!). I cried and felt so many things in that moment: joy, fear, hope, gratitude, surprise.

Once my 5 minutes of disbelief and incredulity had passed, I texted my husband, asking him to come into the house. I couldn't even talk when he came inside, so I just pointed to the bathroom and let him figure it out. I was going to fall apart if I said the words out loud. He looked at me and asked, "Is it positive?" He was shocked, surprised, and so happy. We hugged and lived in the moment together.

But what was the next thing out of my mouth?!?

"This doesn't mean it will stick."

My earlier miscarriage was a painful reminder that just because I got pregnant, there was no guarantee that I would stay pregnant. I will never forget enduring the pain of that loss, and I think by preparing him for the worst, while reminding myself, maybe I could protect myself from getting too attached, just in case...

All the same, we were going to be parents!

I was finally pregnant! We were so excited and so overwhelmed. We had waited so long for this!!

Jonathan and I happily went to every appointment, together. At the first ultrasound, I had to go back first and endure part of the procedure alone. I was so nervous and scared that we would get bad news. But bad news didn't come. Seeing and hearing our baby for the first time was incredible. I also learned at that appointment that babies will actually react when daddy comes into the room! Did you know that the baby's heartbeat will get stronger when daddy is nearby?

On January 23, 2014, at 10:14 a.m., we welcomed our baby girl into this world. Hearing her cry for that first time was like music to my ears! I was a mommy, after waiting for so long!

A little over a year after our daughter was born, we decided that we wanted to have another baby, in hopes that we would have a little boy. It was a happy time for us even though we didn't know what trying again would be like, considering what we went through to conceive our daughter. We hoped for the best, of course, but we questioned if it would be a challenge again.

We agreed that we would not reach out for help this time and that we would just put it out to the universe that we were ready for another baby. Just a few months later, we were pleasantly surprised to discover we were expecting again! We were so excited because it happened naturally and because it happened so fast!

At my first appointment to confirm the pregnancy, I was very disappointed to find out that while there was a gestational sac, there wasn't a fetal pole. I was having another miscarriage. This was not what we had hoped for, and it was heartbreaking. Having had a miscarriage many years ago, I already knew what it was like to lose a baby, and I was deeply concerned about how I would handle it this time around.

I reached out to a friend, a mom of multiple children, who worked as a doula and was really knowledgeable about pregnancy. She recommended getting a progesterone cream to support my progesterone levels. She also mentioned that I should request for my doctor to check my progesterone levels. With her encouragement, I did some research and learned about how important progesterone is in not only conceiving, but also in maintaining a pregnancy.

At my next appointment, I needed more blood work done and requested that my doctor check my progesterone. Though my OB said that wasn't a normal part of the blood work for this, citing that "progesterone isn't an important factor in pregnancy," she agreed to it after I firmly insisted.

TIP: If you feel that there is something wrong or that doctors are missing something in their evaluation, tests, or diagnosis, DO NOT be afraid to push them to do more evaluations and tests. It is your body and your care. Trust your gut.

The test showed that my progesterone levels were indeed pretty low. In my opinion, we lost our second child to miscarriage because of low progesterone levels. This was hard on me, and I felt alone in the process. My husband was caring for our toddler and wasn't able to comfort me through the worst moments. This time, however, the loss didn't hit me as hard as the first had; I think that was because I had a child to care for and maybe because I was able to mentally prepare myself due to my previous loss.

If you have ever suffered through the loss of a pregnancy, you know the mental battle that comes along after that loss.

What did I do wrong?

Why did this happen to me?

What could I have done differently?

Want to know something? It wasn't my fault, and it isn't yours either. I have heard it said that there is little you can do to cause or prevent the loss of a baby. In most cases, it is your body detecting a problem and aborting the process often before you even know it has begun.

Our doctor recommended waiting 6 months before trying again; however, we started trying almost right away. The one thing I did differently this time was supporting my progesterone balance with a natural serum, and I started this as soon as I knew I was losing our baby in the summer.

We conceived again, right around Christmas, and knowing that I was doing what my body had needed me to do, I was sure this time would be different. This pregnancy was healthy, uneventful, and went to term; he was even born at home.

When we know better, we do better!

Today, we have four children and never needed help conceiving after conceiving our first pregnancy through IUI. Never give up on your dreams; know that the desire on your heart to be a mom was put there by God, and He will fulfill that desire. It may look different than what you imagined, and your journey may take twists and turns that you didn't think possible. Keep the faith and trust in His word. Your time is coming!

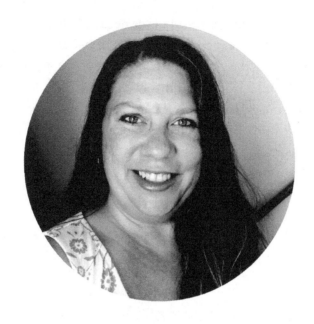

Scan the code for a video message from Amanda and a free gift

Amanda Ignot is a wife, mother, entrepreneur, and natural birth coach. She currently lives in Columbia, Missouri, with her husband and four children. She lives to educate and empower women on their pregnancy and childbirth journeys giving them back their power to envision the birth they truly are capable of. Her journey to motherhood was not an easy one, and yet she overcame the hard times, kept going, and had beautiful experiences along the way. Today, you may find her traveling across the country, with her children in tow, to attend the birth of a friend and accomplish her goals.

https://amandaignot.com/page/links

YEARS OF INFERTILITY-ANGER, SADNESS, DISAPPOINTMENT, MIRACLES, AND EVEN A GIRL NAMED HOPE

Cindy D. Vochatzer-Murillo

love, love, love stories and the people in them, so I am going to share my story with you. It is a story of despair, hope, sadness, disappointment, miracles, and even a girl named Hope.

My story begins in childhood. I thought when I was a child that I would finish high school, go to college, begin dating, and find the man of my dreams, marry, start a family, and become a mom. It would be just like the Disney fairytale.

Well, it didn't happen like that in OUR story.

My story is 12 years of meandering through life, including seven years of infertility.

A few months shy of my 30th birthday, my husband and I decided that we would stop using any birth control. I had been on birth control for more than 8 years, but I was never the best about remembering to take the pill at the same time every day. Sometimes I would miss days, but I never found myself accidentally pregnant. You can't take the pill wrong more times than right and not find yourself pregnant. That should've been the first clue that I had a struggle ahead of me.

At that time, my cycles were regular, but longer than the normal 21-28 days. One month, my period stopped, I went to the doctor. I needed to find out why. My OB/GYN did some blood work. The labs came back saying that my testosterone levels were *four times* higher than they should be in women, and my progesterone levels were low. They diagnosed me with polycystic ovarian syndrome, otherwise known as PCOS. The doctor told me that 1 in 10 women have it. Not rare but not very common either.

After my diagnosis, when I talked about PCOS in a room of 10 women, 9 would have the diagnosis. My thought is either doctors are over-labeling PCOS or it's not really a 1 in 10 issue. We struggled for many more years with me cycle tracking and testing daily for my ovulation. In the end, it was pointless because of my PCOS; I never got a positive test for ovulation. (This information is now included on the side of ovulation test kit boxes.)

In the end, the doctor said the only way to balance my hormones was to stay on the birth control pill. Huh! It's hard to conceive when you are on the pill. I felt like the doctors didn't know what they were talking about. These confusing statements set me on a journey of questioning everything. I began to ask why over and over again until I got answers or understanding.

From that moment on, I took 100% ownership over my health and my body. I looked into what I was putting in and on my body. I quit drinking soft drinks, and that was so hard since everyone around me drank pop, but I realized that soft drinks are just as addictive as drugs and alcohol. I would experience withdrawals from not getting my soft drink fix. I didn't love the bubbles/carbonation; it was the syrup that tasted so good. I was determined to have a baby, so I was willing to sacrifice and do what it took to wean myself off syrupy soft drinks.

> *TIP: Don't ever start drinking soft drinks, and kick the toxins out of all your personal care products and food. Watch what you put on your body. I put all of that lovely smelly lotion on all through my childhood, and now, we know that the chemicals and toxins in our beauty products contribute to endocrine disruption.*

After my PCOS diagnosis, I had an ultrasound to see how many eggs I had. Turns out I had a lot more on one ovary than the other. In my mind, this is what happens each month. I envision a soft drink machine (funny illustration since I just talked about my journey to give up soft drinks). Each month of my cycle is like putting money into the vending machine and making my selection. One month, the egg drops down into the uterus to be fertilized, and the other month, I put my money in and the machine (my ovaries) thinks it drops the egg, but it doesn't. Because of this, I only had a chance every other month to conceive.

In addition, my ovulation was very late in the month (just a few days before my period started). I don't know why I ovulate like that; it was something I figured out on my own by tracking my cycle. We tried six months of Clomid without success, I was already tired of being poked and prodded, and everything feeling like a science experiment, so IVF wasn't an option at that point.

> *TIP: Build up a strong backbone. You will be in a fight with doctors over who has better knowledge of your body. They may have gone to school for 8+ years, but you have lived in your body longer than that. You are the expert on your health and body.*

We decided to try intrauterine insemination (IUI) one time. I felt very much like a cow on the livestock farm. I know it's weird, but that's what I always thought about when I was doing that procedure. It was probably not the best mindset to have along the way, but it's honestly how I felt. My heart felt sad during this process, and I just wanted to get pregnant naturally and not feel like an inseminated heifer. I was glad for modern medicine, but it made me feel surreal and weird.

The IUI wasn't successful, but I think the procedure ended up being beneficial in my journey. When I went through the IUI, the OB/GYN told me, "Oh, wow, your cervix is very sticky!" I was surprised and unsure if my cervix was supposed to be sticky.

> *TIP: I believe that "unsticking" my sticky cervix contributed to me being able to get pregnant. Talk to your doctor about the possibility this could be affecting you also.*

As I think back on my journey, everyone I met and everything that I was going through was helping me get to where I was in a better place. Maybe you are asking, "Why did we keep going?" I always prayed to the Lord that he would make me a mother.

Another prayer during all of this was I wanted our pregnancy to be a surprise. If you are reading this book, you are struggling with infertility or know someone who is. You know that when you go through infertility, everything is calculation, labs, and tracking, and you literally *know* every single month when your period will happen. You keep track of everything, and every day, you know what is going on with your body and cycle. "Lord, I would like to have a baby **and** be surprised that I was pregnant," was always my prayer.

I was sure this could never happen and said to myself, "I'm just gonna be happy if I get pregnant." But I always deeply wanted to just have a spontaneous pregnancy.

Then one day, I prayed, "Lord, I don't think you want me to be a mother." I was done. I surrendered to the Lord and said, "You don't want me to be a mother, and I am finally okay with that." Little did know my husband was having the exact same conversation with the Lord. By this time, we'd been married 10 years.

> *TIP: Have faith God will get you through all of your journeys in life. Have hope and don't feel hopeless. Find other women on the same journey as you, so you can support each other with friendship on your journeys.*

I don't remember how my sister told me she was pregnant. I'm sure it was over the phone since we live in different states. I think my mom actually told me first in one of those "I have something to tell you, and we are going to keep this between the two of us," kinds of conversations. Anyone else have those kinds of talks with their mom? I was *so* excited for my sister. I don't think my sister was hesitant to tell me, since I always told her that I hoped she didn't have the problems I had conceiving.

Before my sister's baby shower, I went to have my first-ever professional pedicure. I'm sure you're thinking, "Why is an infertility book talking about pedicures?" Well, it's all part of my story, and you never know where the story will take you. Most often, it is to an unexpected place. I went to have my pedicure, and I sat down with my nail tech. She looked very familiar, and I thought to myself, "Where do I know her from?" Turns out I knew her from a job I'd worked a couple years prior. She would come into the store, and I got to know her a bit. Her name was Hope, and I took it as a sign from God that he sent a girl named Hope to help me on my journey of going from hopeless to hopeful.

We chatted a little bit as she worked on my feet. Since I had never gotten a pedicure, I didn't know what to expect. I thought it seemed like she massaged my legs for a very long time, and it seemed really rough to me. She worked on my feet, and if you know anything about the feet, every organ of your body is represented in a different place on the bottom of your feet.

TIP: I truly believe my feet being stimulated helped stimulate my organs and my lymphatic system.

I had a great time celebrating my sister's baby shower. I know a lot of people experiencing infertility don't go to baby showers. I get it. It's really hard, but it was also very healing for me to be able to go and celebrate my sister and her baby. I was very happy for them. As I returned home from my long weekend celebrating my sister and her new baby, I quickly realized that my period hadn't started while I was away like I'd expected. I often had long cycles, so I didn't give it much thought. After a week, I got curious. So, I said, "What the heck? Let me go take a pregnancy test or two." I stuck the test in the little cup of urine for the 1000th time in my life. All of us infertility girls are very accustomed to peeing in a cup.

I had taken so many tests over the years, but this time, it just felt different. I was so nervous waiting for the test to finish. Maybe it was because it was unexpected since I had already surrendered to the Lord and made peace with not being a mom.

Then, I got two pink lines for the first time ever in my life! So, I took another one! I said to myself, "Oh, my goodness, how did I find two faulty pregnancy tests? Crazy! How in the heck did it happen that out of all these tests on the shelf, I picked two broken ones?" I went back to the store and got three more tests because I thought to myself, "You can't possibly find three bad tests." I took each of those, dunked them in my new cup of pee, and the plus signs immediately showed up on each. I thought, "What in the world is happening?! How did I find three more bad pregnancy tests?" I went back to the store for two more, (the expensive ones this time), and got the same result.

I felt nervous, excited, and a little mad since I was suspicious of the results never having had a test come up positive. I waited for my husband to come home from work, and he barely got in the door before I showed him the seven pregnancy tests. He was in shock because we had taken so many tests and had never gotten a positive one. We were in utter disbelief and didn't know what to think or do next.

I decided that I was going to make an appointment with my OBGYN and see what was happening, because I couldn't possibly be pregnant. Luckily, they could get me in by the end of the week. Normally, when I went to the doctor, the first thing they had me do is pee in a cup for a pregnancy test. This time, they didn't do that. Instead, they took me straight into the ultrasound room for a transvaginal ultrasound.

The ultrasound tech asked why I was there that day, and I told her about the seven defective pregnancy tests. I said to her, "I'm here to just have the doctor tell me that I'm not pregnant because I haven't been pregnant for seven years, and I've never had a positive pregnancy test until now."

The tech said, "Oh! I can't find anything here. There's nothing to find." She sent me to a little room to wait on the midwife. I was so confused! They never told me if I was pregnant. The midwife came in and told me that I need to come in every day for the next three days to check my hCG levels to see if they are doubling every 48-hours.

The midwife freaked me out and said if I had any abdominal cramping, to go straight to the emergency room because I could die of a tubal pregnancy. I was like," Whoa, whoa, whoa, let's back up here! We are having all these talks about testing and maybe dying, but nobody has told me if I am pregnant or not!"

The midwife says, "Oh, you're pregnant; we just don't know where the baby is!"

I felt so mad because I had been sitting in the doctor's office for more than two hours, and they had scared me to death thinking I was going to die. I came in to be told that I had seven false positive pregnancy tests. Now, I was being told that I'm pregnant, but they didn't know where the baby was, and I could die this weekend.

They scheduled me to come back in on Monday morning to draw blood and check my hCG levels.

Whew! Let's take that all in. That's a whole bunch of 7 - 12 years of infertility emotions coming all to head as I'm sitting alone in this doctor's office. I didn't take my husband with me because I didn't think I was pregnant. I was convinced I just had some false positive tests.

To make a long story short, I didn't die because I'm here writing this chapter. Turns out, I was very early in my pregnancy, and the doctor's office should have done a urine test first instead of an ultrasound. They should have told me I was pregnant and looked at the calendar to see that I was in that two-week window where you're pregnant, but all the things are happening on a very cellular level, so there's no sac, there's no baby, there's nothing to see. It was not a tubal pregnancy; it was just too early to see our baby.

Because of that traumatic OB/GYN experience, a passion was ignited in me about advocacy for pregnancy, the care of pregnant women, and unborn babies. No woman should stay in the doctor's office by herself and have somebody tell her she could die that weekend (all without saying she is pregnant).

I'm happy to say that after twelve long years of not being able to have a child and seven years of actually trying, our Ellie was born. She's absolutely beautiful. She's our miracle from God. We only have her because of God. *There wasn't anything else that I could have done better or tried harder to have a child.* God gave us this wonderful gift and the story to tell, so others can see that getting pregnant doesn't always happen in our time but in His time.

Three short months after she was born, on August 12th, she was baptized as a child of God. The date just happens to be our 12th wedding anniversary. It was the best anniversary present any couple could ask for. As an added bonus, my sister ended up with two daughters, and Ellie and my nieces are all seven months apart in age. So even though my little sister is four years younger than me, we have kids the same age.

I look back on my infertility journey, and I think that everything happened exactly the way it was supposed to. Remember, I don't believe in any coincidences. There were people and places and opportunities that were placed in front of me. I was supposed to learn new things. The Lord literally picked me to be this older mom.

As I'm writing this, I am a 44-year-old mom to an 8-year-old child. Reflecting on my journey. I wouldn't have been a good mom if I had gotten pregnant when I was 24 and freshly married. I needed more life experience and wisdom. I needed to grow a strong backbone to learn to tell the doctors, "NO, we aren't doing that," to get the pregnancy and delivery I wanted. I was supposed to be an older mom of a young child so I can help other mothers of any age get the pregnancy and delivery they want.

Thank you for reading about my journey. I hope it shows you that you are not alone, and you can do hard things. It is part of your story, just like my journey was part of my story and made me a stronger woman and a stronger mom for my daughter.

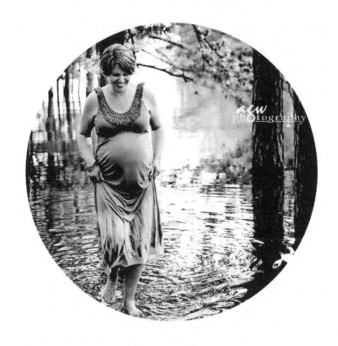

Scan the code for a video message from Cindy and a free gift

Cindy Vochatzer-Murillo is a mom, wife, dog mom, advocate, entrepreneur, course creator and fierce advocate for infertility education. She is a straight shooter that tells it like it is. She currently lives in Atlanta, GA with her husband, daughter and rescue dog Dusty. She is on a mission to help other moms navigate life well through all her life experiences. These experiences have forged her in the fire and she came out the other side sharper than ever. Through these experiences she is able to give moms the easy button and not have the same struggles as her. She loves to read and travel. She has been to several countries and 48 U.S. States with plans to visit the last 2. She also plays a mean game of UNO.

IT'S TIME TO FIRE YOUR OB/GYN!

Amber Stier

I f you're here, you know. You are part of a club you never wanted to be part of and that you likely never knew existed when you started down the path of "womanhood" - I know I didn't.

I started my first period in the sixth grade. It was about as typical as you can get. I went to the nurse's office, and she gave me a pad and Tylenol while I waited for new shorts.

When I got home that evening, I was met with a lot of emotion over a baby girl growing up and not a lot of information. I can't fault my mother; you only know what you know, and she knew *perfectly regular* cycles each month that she tamed with Midol. That wasn't me. My cycles came and went as they pleased. I would mention to the doctors doing my sports physicals that I hadn't had a period in months, and once I assured them that I wasn't sexually active, I was brushed off with, "Oh, that is totally normal for an athlete," or "You are just too [insert stereotype here - thin, active, young] to have a regular period."

Spoiler alert: They were wrong.

Through high school, I was only having periods three to four times per year. I had read that, at 18 years old, women should start seeing an OB/GYN and getting pap smears. Although I wasn't sexually active, I wanted to go because doctors fix things, right? Wrong. Still, "nothing to worry about," "just school stress."

Tip: It is not healthy or normal for your period to be so sporadic. Don't ignore this sign and get it checked out!

During my sophomore year of college, I met my husband, John. We were both at a point in life where we knew what we wanted in a partner, so before we even went on our first date, we talked about kids, dream jobs, places we wanted to live and visit, and even "waiting until marriage" because that was important to us both. Three years later, we married.

Prior to getting married, John and I attended a class at our church to learn NFP or natural family planning. NFP is a form of natural birth control that is based on symptoms like body temperature and cervical mucus. The idea is that if you know when you ovulate, you can either have sex during that time to conceive or not and avoid pregnancy. This method is used by NaPro specialists. Natural procreative technology is an approach to understanding women's reproductive health and regulating fertility by identifying and treating the underlying causes of problems. Why didn't more women know about this and use it? To me, it was empowering to know that women's bodies were so perfectly made, and what was just bleeding each month to me before became a harmony of hormones and follicles and eggs releasing and physical cues. Like a well-oiled machine, it was beautiful, at least for most women it was.

This is where my mission began. It was an attempt to figure out why I wasn't regular. I went to my local OB/GYN to be cured and to choose my own destiny. The first thing my doctor did was an ultrasound. Everything seemed to be as it should except that blood from the missed periods was collecting in the lining of my uterus. He started me on 10 days of progesterone that would trigger a period to shed the old tissue. I did this for the next several months – 10 days of progesterone, 5-7 days of period, 12 days of nothing, repeat progesterone.

I started doing research. Just because I was bleeding each month didn't mean I was ovulating, and ovulation is the FOUNDATION of all the tracking. I was beginning to realize our journey would be different. I was frustrated at my doctor for giving me false periods and, seemingly, not caring enough to fix the reason I wasn't having periods (not ovulating) in the first place.

TIP: Do NOT waste your time with a "regular" OB/GYN. They are really good at treating "normal" people. If you have the slightest inkling, you are abnormal, go straight to a specialist. I will always recommend a NaPro specialist.

About two years into marriage, I hadn't had a period for six months. I knew it was time to go back to the doctor. He started me on the same progesterone protocol. I was frustrated but naively thought that things could have changed in two years. After a few rounds of progesterone to clear out what had been accumulating, he started me on my first round of Clomid.

Even with the forced ovulation using Clomid, my cycles were incredibly long 35-38 days. We tried until we maxed out the dosage. Then we had an HSG (hysterosalpingography). Mine came back normal and clear as all my tests had. The doctor did mention that, due to my history of infrequent cycles and other hormonal issues, I *may* have borderline PCOS (polycystic ovarian syndrome), but he did not have enough information.

In addition to learning about my medications, I began switching out everything - laundry detergent, deodorant, lotion, shampoo. Everything that went *on* my body was scrutinized.

Soon after I started the journey of cleaning up my household products, I learned about essential oils and what they could do for women's hormones. I came across a book which had a "troubleshooting" guide. There were protocols for typical issues: amenorrhea, short cycles, and for me - long cycles! I started following this protocol. I went from almost 40-day cycles down to 28–30-day cycles. And then, it happened. In August 2015, we had our first positive pregnancy test.

We had been married four years at that point. I remember taking the test and coming back to a faint second line. I sat there on the floor, begging for it to be real. There was no cutesy, planned-out surprise to tell my husband. I couldn't wait. I ran directly to him and said, "It's positive." We were both in disbelief. I called my doctor's office, and they said, "Great, see you at eight weeks." That felt like an eternity. Thankfully, I worked for a company that had its own clinic. When I told them of the pregnancy, they did a blood HCG and progesterone level test so that we could make sure everything was increasing as it should.

Before I got the test results back, we left on summer vacation. The weekend was perfect. John and I were on cloud nine the entire time. We went out to eat and took a picture together, and that was the first picture of the "3" of us. Sometimes, I look back at that picture and stare into my eyes. That version of me had never experienced loss before. She still believed that a positive pregnancy test equaled a baby to hold and to love in nine months.

Monday morning came, and I got a phone call. "Your numbers are going down instead of up. We believe you are having a 'chemical pregnancy' and that you will likely start your period soon." And I did. I had never bled so much nor felt so empty in my life. Loss #1.

At my next appointment, my doctor asked if I had done anything different in order to conceive. I described "cleaning up" my routine, not sure how he would react. Surprisingly, he responded with, "Well, it seems to be working. So, I guess, keep doing it." So, I did. And in February, we had another positive test.

I was guarded and cautiously optimistic. My HCG numbers went up from the initial draw. It was very little, but up, not down. Because of this increase and my history, I was scheduled for an ultrasound. When the day came, my worst fears were realized. "I can't find a heartbeat, and what is supposed to be in your uterus is not in your uterus." I was reeling.

The next couple of hours were a blur. I met my doctor at his office. "Your pregnancy is ectopic. You can either go get two shots of Methotrexate at the cancer center, or we can get you into surgery right now. You aren't leaving here until we do one of those two things." I called my husband, and we agreed that since there was no longer (or maybe never was) a heartbeat, that we would preserve my tube and do the shots.

John offered to drop everything and come be with me, but I refused. I'm not sure if I was trying to be "Miss Independent" or if I was just trying to protect him. I did that a lot during our journey, not to intentionally keep information from him, but at the time, I thought it would be easier on him if I carried all the burden.

> *TIP: Include your husband in as much as he is comfortable, not only to relieve yourself of some of the burden, but it's also important for his processing and healing.*

I arrived at our local cancer center. They brought me back, gave me the shots, and I left. Loss #2.

It was time to move on. At my next appointment, I asked if I could be referred elsewhere. He said that while they usually don't refer out until after a minimum of three losses, he was "willing" to go ahead and do it because there wasn't any more, he could do for me.

> *Tip: Advocate for yourself. Don't waste time with people who won't work with you and just continuously put you through all the "normal" protocols.*

My first appointment with a fertility specialist was in April. Because we had been pregnant before, he thought he could help us. I left that appointment with renewed hope. He put me on Metformin and an extra 500 mg of folate in addition to what was in my prenatal vitamin. While I was still diagnosed as "unexplained infertility," Metformin helps balance blood sugar and is a common drug used in patients with PCOS.

Before we could get started on this plan, I was pregnant again in May. We did the usual tests, and the numbers were low. By this time, my heart was so covered with calluses that I was prepared. I didn't need to get the second blood draw. I knew. One good thing about all of this - you get to know your body really, really well. The numbers declined, and soon after, I started my period. Loss #3.

We took tests – karyotyping and a panel of blood clotting disorders. Karyotyping is where they check the DNA of the partners to make sure they can align properly and that there isn't a genetic reason for the recurrent miscarriages. Our results came back normal. The results for my clotting panel came back normal or negative on all types except for the MTHFR (methylenetetrahydrofolate reductase) gene mutation. I have one copy (hetero) C677T. It is said that this type is "unlikely to be of clinical significance."

TIP: Get these tests done early on. You never know what you will find, and managed clotting disorders can prevent devastating miscarriages!

At this point, I had had my fair share of pelvic ultrasounds, but in July, the stars aligned to give me a real diagnosis. On this day 4 ultrasound, the doctor made a not reassuring, "Huh, look at that" comment. He moved the wand around to show me the several circles amid the black background of the ovary. "It's called a pearl necklace," he said. I'm sure the look on my face said it all. "Cysts that form a circle on the ovaries. It is a tell-tale sign of PCOS," he explained.

After five years of "unexplained infertility," I finally got my diagnosis of PCOS. I now had a name and a face to the monster. Nothing changed in my treatment, but my insurance company would believe it and help pay to keep it in check.

In August, after a Letrozole (Femera) induced ovulation, I got another positive home pregnancy test. By this time, I had my routine down. I go in for my blood test. HCG - low, progesterone - decent. However, as I went through my day, I knew this wasn't a lasting pregnancy. Less than two weeks after I got the positive test, I started to miscarry. Loss #4.

Life kept on moving. We had purchased a new house earlier in the summer, and I left my job shortly after. I was so broken and felt like a failure. We had celebrated our fifth wedding anniversary and were recovering from our fourth miscarriage. Who was this person I had become? She wasn't the blissfully happy mom of four children (two girls and two boys, of course) that I had imagined. Thankfully, I had my husband to hold me up. I've heard that marriage is rarely 50/50. Often, one spouse or the other is going through something that requires the other to take on more. This was my husband during a time when I was falling apart and asking, "I did everything in the right order, God; why am I being punished? Why are people that are doing everything out of order and have broken homes having children and not me?"

TIP: Give yourself some grace; these triggers will happen. You choose how you react to them.

Have you ever seen each step that God placed for you to get through a storm? Soon after this loss, a friend invited me to a Bible study, where another woman and I became fast friends. It became clear quickly that we had a lot in common, including infertility. She told me the doctor she was working with specialized in NaPro technology. The dots from all those years ago connected at that Bible study. I just wish I had listened earlier!

I didn't hesitate to call and make an appointment. The NaPro method was appealing because 1. Its intention was to get to the root of the issue and 2. We are devout in our practice of Catholicism and always felt like we needed to be on high alert for any medicine or procedure that would not align with the teachings of the church. When we found this NaPro practitioner, we felt the weight lift off of us because the premise comes from working *with* the nature and dignity of a woman's body to help it do what it was naturally meant to do. We never felt uneasy or like we had to question the morality of it.

Our first appointment with the NaPro specialist was eye-opening. She agreed with the PCOS diagnosis but wanted to check my thyroid and have John tested. Believe it or not, *no other doctor* had mentioned a sperm analysis! She also suggested that we have a consultation and possible laparoscopic surgery to check and rule out endometriosis.

TIP: Even if you don't think the issue is your husband, get him checked too. Male factor is more prevalent than you think!

Don't be afraid to get an early lap to check for endometriosis. It is not visible on scans and is a major player in infertility. Typical symptoms include cramps during your period and pain during sex.

The thyroid panel came back saying I was a bit low, and we made our appointment for the laparoscopic surgery. John's results came back normal as well, and now, we knew.

In addition to the tests, I started a slew of new vitamins and supplements. It was not my favorite thing to do - taking so many pills at certain times of the day and with or without food. But I was hopeful and willing to try what she recommended. It was also about this time that I forced myself to start a workout routine. I hadn't done anything on a regular basis since high school! I loved it and hated it at the same time.

A few months later, we went out of town, and when we returned, I realized I had missed my Letrozole for that month. I was upset, but nothing could be done. Nevertheless, we tried a couple of times just in case!

As soon as I was late, I took a test. I was using the digital Clearblue tests and will never forget seeing "Pregnant" on the screen. There was no fanfare. I immediately took the test to John and said, "Well, here we go again."

We called that day and got in for the usual blood tests. I started doing daily Lovenox injections and oral progesterone. The numbers looked good, and so did the second draw numbers. We went to the office for our first ultrasound. There it was: the *heartbeat*. John and I met eyes. It was the first one we had ever seen. It was beautiful and perfect, and I was completely awestruck by the miracle of it.

During that appointment, I also had my first progesterone injection. I continued those throughout pregnancy, along with my prenatal vitamin, Lovenox injections daily, LDN - low dose Naltrexone, Armour Thyroid, a low dose (81mg) aspirin, 500mg folate and Ovasitol.

It is difficult to explain the feelings we had. Each day was a miracle, yet we were on eggshells the entire time. Overall, the pregnancy went well, and we were blessed with an amazing baby boy at exactly 40 weeks. He is perfect in every way. There are a few things I would have done differently, and they are contained in the tips above.

TIP: Above all, fire your regular OB/GYN early and advocate for all the testing.

Thanks to the bravery of the women in this book, I pray your journey is much shorter, sweet sister!

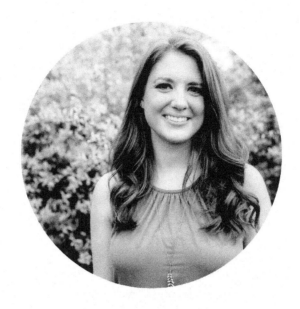

Scan the code for a video message from Amber and a free gift

Amber was born and raised in southeastern Indiana. Growing up, she never imagined that infertility would be part of her life's story. She is wife to John and, through the blessing of NaPro, is mother to one wild, miracle boy. Together, they enjoy a slow-paced life in the country and often capitalize on the fact that they live close to family. When they are not spending time with family, the three of them escape to hike and camp in Michigan as often as possible. *Infertility Success* is her first book, and she hopes it will help many women shorten their infertility journey.

msha.ke/amberstier

THE SCARS OF JOY

Jacci Robyn Lötter

Four biological children and two adopted.

I had a plan.

I dreamed of a large family … family lunches, kids playing in the house, family being part of each other's lives … big, loud, messy, and happy.

Life made other plans for me when I wasn't watching, though, and my perfect plan hung in the balance because of severe PCOS and insulin resistance, sporadic cycles, and tons of pain.

With the patience of Job, my husband supported my dreams of having a family. All these challenges only further fueled my pit-bull-like stubbornness to have what I had dreamed about, so after a few years of marriage, we began receiving fertility treatment through our OB/GYN, and finally fell pregnant. Clomid was my friend!

Our happy ending had begun.

With the eagerness of any young mother, I attended our 12-week scan with an already bulging belly which could only be contained by maternity clothing.

Where there were previously twins, there were now no heartbeats... They called it a "missed abortion," as if anything could describe it more horrendously.

I was required to take one single tablet which expels "a foetus" from its mother. It had cost thousands to achieve a pregnancy but less than 50 cents for this one tablet which would end it all.

I was in shock as we prepared for me to have an evacuation the next day. I still had overwhelming morning sickness, and I could not compute how this was happening.

Foetus. Evacuation. Missed abortion. All words which get thrown around to describe your child, your future. It was all so cold.

Despite the heartache after our loss, we tried again almost immediately. We seemed to have found what worked to get me pregnant, but it soon became clear that Clomid was not the magic bullet we had hoped for as I had miscarriage after miscarriage, bleeding out more hope each time.

I was seven weeks pregnant again, and I felt a familiar gush. The warm blood was soaking my clothes. I was hemorrhaging clots down my pantihose.

Despite my history and what was going on in my body, I felt in my soul that, somehow, this baby was here to stay.

This one was going to be the one I held in my arms. I'd prayed, and it was confirmed in a way I could not deny, even as I was sitting on a plastic grocery store bag, trying not to soak the car seat in blood.

The ER doctor confirmed that my cervix was, in fact, closed, and there was still a heartbeat! The joy I felt was immeasurable. This felt a little like hope. I was put on strict bed rest for the first trimester, though I continued to hemorrhage every few days. Every time I bled; I was left wondering if this was the final gush … if this was the clot which was actually my baby leaving my body.

Following a particularly large bleed, Dr. M., a stand-in for my regular OB/GYN, took one look at my pale face and, without examining me, said, "By the looks of you, we will probably schedule you for an evacuation tomorrow." I looked at her in absolute disgust and demanded the scan. *How DARE she* make such an assumption? As I predicted, there was still a heartbeat, and I vowed that Dr. M. would never touch me or my baby again. I needed people around me who were willing to fight for my child's life.

Mercifully, the bleeding stopped by the second trimester through use of high doses of progesterone and bedrest, and we were able to breathe again as we found out we were having a little girl.

We finally got to use the name we had carefully chosen within the first month of our marriage … *Chloë*.

The injections, scans, terrible progesterone suppositories which clogged up every orifice … It was all going to be worth it.

But our bliss was short-lived as I started developing preeclampsia by 17 weeks.

By 22 weeks, our little girl was very small.

Too small.

As luck would have it, Dr. M. was on call again and delivered the report of Chloë's health over the phone. My stomach was bursting with life and movement as our little girl wriggled while we spoke.

Without regard for my journey (or the fact that I was a human being), Dr. M. coldly said, "Jacci, I hope you didn't get your hopes up about this pregnancy. The foetus will not survive, but you are young, so you can try again."

When I asked if there wasn't SOMETHING we could try, she offered me no hope.

The **mother** in me was birthed in that moment.

I got second opinions, called in every favor I could, prayed, and asked family and friends to fast for us. If there was anything in this world which could be done, I wanted to know about it, and I didn't rest until I felt we had a solid plan.

While the prognosis wasn't great, there WERE things I could do.

I was placed on strict bedrest again with fistfuls of medication, monitoring my blood pressure three times a day, and having scans every few days to check on her.

After the latest incident with Dr. M., I called up my OB/GYN to tell her I would no longer accept Dr. M. on my medical team. Another doctor was arranged for emergencies, but my OB/GYN made herself available to me a lot more than usual too. I realized that I had to emphatically state what my boundaries were, so they were not crossed again.

From then on, a team of people were called in for additional counsel. We would utilize the collective expertise of many doctors, who were also invested in **saving** *Chloe's* life.

TIP: Remember that you are paying medical experts to help you on your journey. It is not THEIR journey, and you are their customer. Find someone else if their ethos does not

> *align with yours. Get recommendations for doctors from friends or online forums. Never feel bad to have your records transferred.*

It was clear that Chloë would be born prematurely. My dreams of a natural birth evaporated as she was too small and fragile to endure labor or travelling through the birth canal. But she would be safer, and I made my peace very quickly.

My view was that birth is an event. Health is for a lifetime. While I appreciate that it is not always so simple, I had to establish in my mind that the birth I **wanted** was not what she **needed**. Mom face on; C-section, here we come.

Despite being vocal about our desire to do everything possible to increase her odds of survival, we were offered an abortion just two days before her scheduled birth. I raged, instructing the pediatrician that if he was not prepared to fight for her, I would find someone who would. I was prepared, at that moment, to shuffle the entire NICU and OB/GYN team to find care providers who would rise up for us.

I may have been young, but I was fierce, and they needed to match my passion, or they would need to make way for someone who would.

Chloë's birth was very traumatic for me. Waking up in pain, not knowing if my daughter was alive, was the scariest thing I had ever endured. As soon as I was vaguely conscious, I was wheeled into the NICU to meet her – the tiniest, most beautiful little girl, weighing only 460 grams.

She was so small, covered in tubes. But she was my whole life's purpose.

As the weeks went on, we were the happiest we had ever been. Parenting, even in the NICU, was the best feeling of our lives. Chloë was a feisty, pretty baby girl who filled us with joy.

Though she was small, she was mighty, and she was the love of our lives.

We knew everything about her care, and my mother's instinct was in full force. By week three, I could tell the nurses how far to insert the ventilator. We were in sync with Chloë and knew her medical needs almost better than the nurses. In hindsight, I wish I'd trusted that gift more.

TIP: TRUST your instinct. A mother KNOWS. At worst, you are overprotective, and at best, you could save your child's life. I believe mother's intuition is a God-given POWER, which no doctor can match or quantify. The more you trust that power, the more it will work for you.

One day, when Chloë was five weeks old, she stopped breathing for a minute when I was holding her. Once stable, I asked the nurses to take more blood tests to make sure she was okay, but they didn't want to prick her for nothing. The thought of hurting her for no reason silenced me.

Two days later, I gasped for air through my sobs, as I held my miracle baby for the last time. Our precious Chloë, the one who had made us parents, died in my arms.

My dreams of being a mother were shattered more cruelly than I ever imagined possible. Why had I not insisted on those blood tests? The thought haunts me to this day.

There are no words to describe the loss, guilt, or the physical and emotional pain of being parents with empty arms after having them filled ever so briefly.

Walking out of that NICU with no baby, my husband told me through sobs that he never wanted another child. He just wanted her back.

Fortunately, the very next day, we both realized that parenthood was worth fighting for again. Chloë would always be ours.

Our world had been rocked, and we were forever changed.

I was able to try to fall pregnant again five months after Chloë's death. The break was, in part, because I needed to wait for my scars and uterus to heal before another pregnancy, but also, our psychologist advised that I needed to heal emotionally first. My body was a WRECK, and my husband needed me to work through everything happening in our lives. He wanted his wife to be okay because I was all he felt he had left. My psychologist encouraged me to change jobs, which was amazing advice. Working with a passion of mine helped give me strength to endure further treatments.

TIP: Having a skilled professional to counsel you through infertility and loss is the single most impactful thing one can do to navigate the trauma of loss. Healing is deeply amplified.

You will not resonate with every counsellor. Find one you connect with deeply.

Shop around!

When we started trying again, we moved to a fertility specialist who was more equipped to deal with our case, and immediately, one problem was solved. A simple procedure to check for a uterine septum was recommended immediately; I had a **massive** one.

It seems that each lost pregnancy had attached to it, and with the restricted blood flow, the babies could not grow.

While Chloë had attached to a healthy site, the septum eventually stunted her growth, and the bleeding may have been the result of the placenta breaking away from where it was growing on the septum.

Once the septum was removed in a completely painless and quick procedure, keeping a pregnancy would be easier.

TIP: After experiencing challenges with conception, go straight to a fertility specialist. An OB/GYN is not an expert in putting babies inside you. They are experts in getting them OUT of you.

Following an ectopic pregnancy, on Mother's Day 2011, I awoke sick with the flu while on my umpteenth round of treatment with injections and insemination.

This would be the last one.

Our finances were drained, and I was worn and battered from life in general, but at that moment, it was the flu kicking my butt.

I decided to take a pregnancy test, and if it was negative, I was going to pound the flu meds. If anything, good could come from what I was sure would be a negative test, it would be that I could finally take some medication to relieve my flu symptoms.

But I was PREGNANT.

I read that screen over and over.

The flu got frightened away faster than a toddler's tantrum at the sight of candy as I ran to the bedroom and waved a urine-soaked stick in my sleeping husband's face.

The pathologists opened especially for me that Sunday morning for a blood test; they all knew my journey, and through the hundreds of blood tests I'd had through them, they were heavily invested in my reproductive ventures.

On what was going to be my second Mother's Day without Chloë, Mother's Day took a turn in a wonderful direction because I was pregnant with TWINS!

Previously, all our baby dreams had been in pink with Chloë, and as this pregnancy progressed, it felt surreal to be dreaming in pink AND blue!

Our little girl would be named Addison, and our son would be named Logan. My belly was almost as full as my heart.

At one of our many scans, we learned that our little girl was sick.

All of the torture endured in that room was coming back from previous scans which ended in tragedy.

Our little Addison had a chromosomal abnormality, and her heart was already struggling.

Because of the potential risk an unhealthy twin has on a healthy twin, we were encouraged to consider selective abortion to give our little boy the best chance of survival.

I was flabbergasted and could not fathom making that choice. It would break me beyond repair.

I was unable to eat or sleep as the decision loomed over us, praying for a miracle for Addison. I knew what a child of that size looked like outside the womb, that they feel pain, and love. I heaved at the prospect of losing her or being forced to end her life to save Logan's.

A week later, we had a scan to check on her, but I think I already knew.

The left side of my stomach was quieter now.

Our doctor scanned me repeatedly ... delivering the devastating news that Addison's heart had stopped.

I was GUTTED that my little boy no longer had his sister, that we had lost another daughter.

My heart broke in a million pieces for Logan and then for my husband, who so badly wanted to have a daddy's girl, but at the same time, I was so grateful to have been spared being the one to make an impossible choice. If she had to die, I was grateful it was like this and not with pain inflicted at her mother's hand.

I was a walking baby coffin. My little Addison would be inside me until her brother was born.

Crying over Addison, we decided we would focus all our attention on Logan.

This pregnancy was now HIS. Another piece of me had died with Addison. I would let that piece of my heart be covered with beautiful flowers and greenery as I devoutly tended to the rest of the garden in my heart, which now belonged to Logan.

We would make sure that whatever happened, he would know he was DEEPLY loved.

We knew we would not be doing this again – Logan was going to be our only child.

From the moment Logan was born, I was in love. He was exactly what I wanted and needed, and I was now able to enjoy my rainbow baby.

The night feeds were amazing and bonded us as we looked into each other's eyes. I knew that he was my person, and he knew I was his. It's always been that way with us.

The scars inside me changed how I mothered him.

Perhaps without them, I would not have enjoyed those midnight feeds as much, or how much I got to hold him when he was colicky.

The innocence of new parthood had been stolen, and not one single day went by that we didn't appreciate having this little boy; it took years for us to not feel like we could lose him at any moment.

We were finally whole again.

From when Logan was four years old, he prayed nightly for a baby brother or sister. We taught him that sometimes, God says, "No," because we needed to protect his faith.

But He *prayed* it into being when my heart was too guarded to ask out loud. We got a surprise "freebie" positive pregnancy test!

This time around, despite my doctor's wishes, I refused weekly scans, and I didn't inject myself. I needed the clean slate for this pregnancy, unmarred by the bad juju of all the losses of the past.

This time, I needed to try and be as normal as possible because all those extra things were going to steal joy again.

> *TIP: Look inward. Is it going to be good for you to have a lot of medical intervention with each pregnancy? Will it settle your mind to feel you are doing all you can, or will it cause you anxiety? You need to advocate for yourself. Your needs may change over time, but always take care of your heart.*

Only when we found out his gender did I start to believe our little boy would be a take-home baby. It felt miraculous that we had another full-term baby.

When Cole arrived in the world, so did we. We were fulfilled in every way.

We would never experience daughters in this life, but my picture was perfect, and I loved so hard, harder than I knew possible.

My obviously unfounded fear of not being able to love another child like I loved Logan and Chloë vanished. Our boys moved us into a space in life where we even forget the struggle sometimes. We'll never forget our babies, but the struggle became mercifully fuzzy.

We feel hope again; through scars, we found our joy.

My dreams from my youth of having four biological children materialized with two daughters in Heaven and two sons on Earth.

One day, our son's wives will be our other two children.

ALL my children are mine, forever and always.

Everything is as it should be, always.

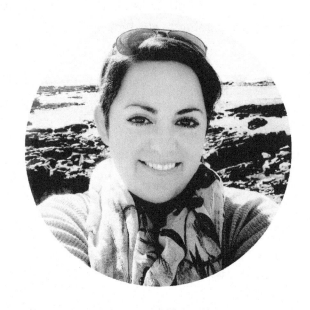

Scan the code for a video message from Jacci and free gift

Jacci Lötter hails from Cape Town, South Africa, and is wife to an architect husband, mother of two beautiful sons on Earth and seven babies in Heaven. Jacci is well acquainted with heartache, loss and, most importantly, immense gratitude.

A strong proponent of highlighting and normalizing hidden challenges such as depression, infertility, and autoimmune diseases, Jacci works with people daily to educate in using natural wellness to get reprieve from previous physical and emotional limitations.

Jacci is a certified life coach and psychology and industrial psychology graduate, focused on upskilling others and leading them to realize their highest potential through mindset, the law of attraction and being one's own advocate.

A lover of education, Jacci has been in the learning and development space in her 15-year career, while also being heavily involved in helping families to have children through her association with big hearted women in the infertility industry.

WHALE SONGS

Drew Jacobs

Where's your dream vacation? That place you've always wanted to go? The place that would be a life-changing experience? Ours was New Zealand and Australia.

My husband, Alex, and I decided to ring in the new year down under.

Then we thought … "Wouldn't it be *amazing* if that was the moment, we started trying to make a baby?" We had it all planned out. Have a once in a lifetime trip across the world and come back pregnant. It couldn't be more magical.

I knew it would be easy. I was young. My mom had no issue conceiving. And I had a nurse tell me during an ovarian ultrasound, "You should be careful. You're *really* fertile." It would be a cinch.

December 27th, we took a 24-hour trip across the world. We spent the next three weeks exploring and "doing it" … a lot. I bought this stuffed kangaroo with a tiny joey in its pouch for our baby. I imagined telling my future child, the one fertilizing that moment in my uterus, the story of "when you were conceived."

A week after we get home, my period arrived.

Huh, that's too bad. I guess we'll keep trying?

The next month came and went. So did the next. And the next.

I started using ovulation kits. The one where the smiley face pops up when it's "go time." I become compulsive with checking my cycle, tracking everything. When the timing seemed "perfect," I jumped on my husband. It's as romantic as it sounds. Still, nothing happened.

I started to develop racing "what if" thoughts in my head. "What if the test is wrong?" "What if I'm not ovulating?" "What if there's something wrong with me?" The thoughts became compulsive. The stress and worry swelled up and crashed down like a wave of disappointment each month.

Then, life took a detour.

During this time, as I'm laser focused on trying to conceive, my sister, Cara, is struggling with an undiagnosed illness. After weeks of testing, we receive an answer – lung cancer.

The following months are a blur. She received treatment, she was in and out of the hospital, and we took turns looking after my niece. At the same time, I was traveling for work as a corporate facilitator. I was coaching people to be present and authentic when inside I was *barely hanging on*.

And every month, I peed on that stick until I saw that stupid smiley face. And every month, my period came.

I don't know why I was still trying at this point. Wouldn't a normal person stop while they're going through this amount of stress? Wouldn't a pregnancy just add an additional layer of anxiety during this time when I need to be there for my family?

I didn't care. I kept going.

Maybe it was something that I felt like I could control. Maybe I was witnessing my sister's life being completely altered, and in some twisted way, I wanted to try to force my own destiny, when the real joke is that the last thing you can control is life.

That July, my creative, funny, ambitious sister passed away.

The best way I can describe how I felt during those first few months with Cara gone was like my whole body was a skinned-knee. You know that feeling when you skin your knee, and the skin is so raw that if the wind blows on it, it stings? It was like that ... but all over.

The months went by, and I was still continuing to try. And I still saw no results. This just exacerbated my grief. It was as if I was carrying around a backpack full of bricks, and as each month went by, another brick was added.

Then, I arrived at the one-year mark, the moment when you're outside of the "normal" time range to conceive, the moment when many insurance companies go, "okay, you've proved you're broken. We'll cover infertility treatment."

We had our initial consultation, where our doctor explained that they'll do a series of tests with the hope of finding out why I couldn't conceive.

I remember walking out of the office feeling completely defeated. "I feel like I failed," I said to Alex. I officially couldn't do it on my own.

I remember the excitement of getting my next period. When you're receiving fertility treatment, your period is a big deal. On one hand, it's another month filled with tears, wine, and sushi. And on the other hand, it's the kick-off to the next phase.

I went through my testing, and I anxiously waited to hear if they "found the reason." We revisited our doctor, and she shared our results: Alex, normal. Drew, normal.

Normal? What does that mean?

It means I have "unexplained infertility." Unexplained infertility is "the lack of an obvious cause for a couple's infertility and the female's inability to get pregnant after at least 12 cycles of unprotected intercourse."

In layman's terms - it means "we don't know what's wrong with you."

Because of my age and health, my doctor recommended an intrauterine insemination (IUI). This was a much less invasive process than IVF.

Everything suddenly felt so exciting. Things were moving. There was momentum.

We went through our first IUI. No results. Then another. No results. We did this a total of four times with no luck.

During this time, months are flying by. My social media is littered with pregnancy announcements. People who conceived their children *after* we started trying are now celebrating their first birthdays. I'm feeling negative and pessimistic, something that is the opposite of who I am.

But I was determined.

Our next option was IVF.

My doctor explained the process:

1. You start with a cycle of the birth control pill.
2. Once your period arrives, you begin monitoring: blood work and an ultrasound to measure your follicle growth. This happens about every other day.
3. You introduce shots – one every night to help multiple follicles grow instead of just one.
4. Then, you add another shot, one that prevents you from ovulating the follicles.
5. When the time is right, you take your "trigger shot," a shot that tells your body it's time to ovulate. Thirty-six hours later, they perform an "egg retrieval," where they retrieve as many eggs as they can that they then fertilize with sperm.

The whole process takes about 2-3 weeks.

It became a big ritual for us. Alex would prepare the shots while I cleaned my abdomen. He would always administer the shots because I was too scared to do it myself.

I went into the office every other day for my monitoring. Each day, I would be filled with anticipation. "Are they growing?" "Are there a lot of them?" The rest of the day, I would hover by the patient portal, waiting for my results to come in. It's a miracle I got any work done.

There are a lot of challenging things about infertility – the disappointment, the cost, the effects of the medication on your body. But what I found most difficult was the unpredictability.

It felt there was no rhyme or reason to anything. Some bodies respond great to meds; some respond poorly. Your cycle can be right on schedule one month, then decide to speed up the next. Each month, I would plan for what could possibly happen, so I wouldn't be distraught by the bad news. And no matter what I prepared for, there was always another surprise around the corner.

One thing you can't plan for is the date of your egg retrieval.

Mine was the day before Thanksgiving. You're not allowed to wear anything on your body except for a pair of socks. A fun ritual many women do is pick out special socks for the day. Mine were these thick, purple, wooly socks. Purple was Cara's favorite color.

That day, they retrieved 12 eggs. I was thrilled with the results. Our baby was one of those eggs!

I woke up Thanksgiving morning feeling on top of the world. I'm sore from the procedure, but I don't care. I curl up with a heating pad and watch the parade. Then, my phone rang.

It was a doctor calling me. His tone was short as if he had limited time and patience for this call, "Your eggs didn't fertilize naturally overnight. In order to still have a chance, we need to do an emergency ICSI (pronounced ick-see). Do I have your permission to do it?"

I was in shock. I started asking him questions. He grew more impatient. "The longer we wait to do this, the less of a chance they'll fertilize. Do I have your permission?"

I said yes, and he hung up.

I had no idea what just happened. I Googled ICSI. It stands for intracytoplasmic sperm injection. It's a process where they take an individual sperm from the sample and directly inject it into the egg.

TIP: Many clinics automatically include ICSI. When investigating treatment centers, ask if this is something they will incorporate.

I chose to shove my anxiety into the back of my head and try to enjoy my Thanksgiving.

The next day, they called me to share that eight of my eggs had been fertilized. I felt an overwhelming sense of relief and hope. Later in the day, they called to schedule a 3-day transfer. It felt like everything was moving in the right direction.

We arrived at the clinic the next day. My bladder was full of water (as instructed), and my whole body was on pins and needles. The room consists of an examination table next to an ultrasound machine. I undressed from the waist down and sat on the edge of the table with a paper sheet wrapped around my lower half.

The doctor and team came in to perform the transfer. All they need is the embryo. The embryologist walks in and says, "Oh, didn't you see the email? I thought we were holding off because it's too early?"

It was another unexpected thing I wasn't prepared for. They postponed my transfer and didn't tell me.

There were many very legitimate reasons why it was postponed, but at that moment, none of them mattered. I sat there, butt on the table, bladder full of fluid, and I softly smiled and said, "It's okay. Thanks for letting me know." When they left the room, I was a puddle of tears in Alex's arms.

I was forced to suck it up and move on to the next stage, a feeling I've realized many women going through this process can relate to.

I waited the remainder of the week to see what embryos made it to the blastocyst stage. Out of the eight, one remained. All of the physical and emotional effort, and I only had one. I was filled with disappointment. But I kept telling myself, "Well, it only takes one, right?"

I began the protocol for my frozen embryo transfer (FET). My process was pretty straightforward. I received monitoring during my cycle, and when the timing was right, they transferred my embryo.

During my whole TTC journey, the one thing I could rely on was my cycle. It was like clockwork. I would always ovulate and menstruate consistently. But this time, something changed. This month, things were delayed. Every monitoring day, I would wait for the call with my transfer date, but every time they called, they would schedule another appointment.

Once we passed the two-week window, I asked, "What's happening? Is my cycle so delayed that I may miss the window to transfer?"

She said, "Yes. There is a chance you may have to wait another month."

It was another moment of unpredictability.

I felt I had gone through so many scenarios in my head of what could happen, but it felt like every time I reached a new stage, another layer of disappointment would be layered in.

During the past few months, I had decided to take up acupuncture. I would see a practitioner named Michelle who was connected to the wellness center at my clinic. She was a really chill, slightly sarcastic woman with a fantastic Scottish accent. She had become a pseudo therapist for me.

I shared through tears that my transfer may be canceled. I'll never forget what she said, "There are a lot of people in my line of work who believe in a higher power. Now, this may all sound like 'whale songs' to you ..." ("whale songs are what she referred to as "woo woo" or "spiritual nonsense") "...but maybe your cycle is delayed for a reason?"

My cycle finally caught up, and I was able to transfer my embryo the day after Christmas. It didn't take.

This meant that if I wanted to keep trying, I had to do another cycle of IVF all over again, something I never thought I would have to do. But what other choice did I have if I wanted to become pregnant?

TIP: Joining an online support group can be helpful in gaining perspective. Hearing multiple stories will broaden your awareness of potential bumps down the road.

This time, I received a different medication protocol to up my follicle count, and they automatically added in ICSI after the retrieval to prevent what happened last time.

I began my second IVF cycle at the beginning of February. This time, I didn't obsess too much about it. I did my own shots since they weren't as scary. And I didn't fixate over the daily doctor's appointments. Thinking back on it, I'm not sure if it was because it felt like old news at this point, or I was trying to emotionally detach from the process, so I wouldn't get hurt.

Because of this, I wasn't paying attention to the calendar. I knew anything could happen at this point. My body might not respond well to the medication, or only two follicles would grow, or my uterus may decide to take a trip to Aruba. Anything was possible.

Then, I got the call. My egg retrieval was set for February 17th. My sister, Cara's, birthday.

I wasn't sure what to think or feel. Is this a good thing or a bad thing? What kind of emotional state would I be in? For me, the birthday of a deceased loved one is dedicated to honoring that person. But with having the egg retrieval that day, I wouldn't be able to celebrate her in the way I wanted.

But then, I had a realization. That day, my eggs, and potentially future children, would be fertilized. It would be the date when their journey began. Essentially, it would be a form of a birthday.

There was the potential that my future child would share a birthday with their Aunt Cara.

On February 17th, they retrieved 17 eggs.

I went to acupuncture and told Michelle this story. She said, "You can believe in 'whale songs' or not, but that happened for a reason. Seventeen eggs on the 17th, which also happens to be your sister's birthday? That's a sign. *That* is why your cycle was delayed. So, it could be on that day."

Out of our 17 eggs, we got four healthy embryos.

We did a fresh transfer five days later. And it didn't take.

Of course, I was devastated. But I was used to bad news at this point. And I had three more embryos to work with.

By this time, I was growing concerned that I may have a deeper issue. My doctor reassured me that she believed I would get pregnant. But she agreed that if the next transfer (which would be my third) wasn't successful, we could investigate further.

TIP: It's okay to advocate for yourself. Although the doctors have the experience, you're one of many patients. Don't be afraid to speak up and make requests.

My third transfer felt like muscle memory, like driving to work or grocery shopping. It wasn't this big emotional moment like the others. Previously, I took the day off and laid on the couch. This time, I drove to work and lived my life as usual.

Five days later, we went to see a play. During the performance, I started to feel cramping. It was the same feeling I get every month before my period – cramping at night and waking up to blood in the morning. As I watched the play, I was internally freaking out.

Driving home, I told Alex, and I completely broke down. For the next hour, I stared out the window, silently sobbing.

I said, "This is the third time it hasn't worked. I *know* there is something going on that we just haven't found yet."

Alex rubbed my leg and said, "You don't know that. It's not over until it's over."

We got home, and me and my puffy, swollen face climbed into bed. With an exhausted whisper, I said to Alex, "Just be prepared for me to have my period tomorrow."

I woke up early. I walked into the bathroom, expecting to discover blood on my toilet paper. And there wasn't any.

I decided to take a test.

And for the first time, in 2 ½ years of trying, the tiniest second pink line appears on the strip. You would think in that moment, there was screaming, crying, and jumping up and down. But all we felt was a quiet, exhilarating sense of relief.

December 28th, my daughter was born. She's named after her aunt, with whom she shares a very special day.

There's a funny thing that happens when you travel from the U.S. across the world. Because of the time change, you actually miss a day when flying. December 27th, when we began our conception journey, we flew from Boston and landed in New Zealand on December 29th. We missed December 28th. Maybe that was some sort of wink from the universe. A spiritual nod telling us that our daughter was coming. Or maybe it's just whale songs. But you know what? I like whale songs.

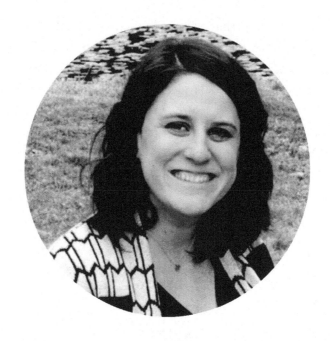

Scan the code for a video message from Drew and a free gift

Drew Jacobs is a mom, wife, sister, and daughter based in Melrose, Massachusetts. She works in the field of leadership development as a facilitator, coach, and instructional designer. She brings her background as a professional actor into her work to help people conquer their communication fears and lead with authenticity. Some of her clients include Harvard Business School, eBay, Prudential Insurance and Pfizer. She loves spending time with her family, cuddling on the couch, and a good hard laugh.

https://linktr.ee/drewjacobs

TRUSTING THE TRAP DOOR

Jules Batchelor

A trap door. Quick sand. A rug pulled out from under me. Hollowness that echoed for weeks. That first loss caught me by surprise. My mother had two easy pregnancies and deliveries. My older sister arrived two years before my twin sister and I were born. My mother had a mother who was horribly tough on her, and we saw the effects. Because of this all, I only ever wanted a chance to be an incredible mom. I wanted a big and happy family.

I was never unaware that to get their struggle was possible, but I was already in my second trimester, having had two successful ultrasounds when it happened. The previous ultrasounds had shown a beautiful little flicker of a heartbeat, which my eyes had become trained to find in the first few moments. I already had two babies- I almost lost the second; but "almost" doesn't matter when you lose one; it only matters that we didn't lose that second one, my beautiful and very extraordinary baby girl. What had started as an exciting appointment to find out the sex (and other important markers) ended with what I now know was as life-changing an experience as I may ever have. I noticed there was no heartbeat before the technician did. My eyes darted around the familiar screen praying for that little blinking pac-man proving a heartbeat. Panic. Panic. PANIC. My toddlers were there wriggling around with the same impatience I was. My (now ex) husband was there. I ordered my family out of the room. I was feeling my eyes sting and blur with tears. I remember being carried, sobbing publicly and shamelessly into my OB/GYN's waiting room.

She scheduled me for a D&C the next day, my body unwilling to expel the baby it was so desperately clinging to. I was given the choice to wait and see if my body would rid the pregnancy naturally, but knowing that it would prolong the pain by potentially waiting (for MONTHS), I opted for immediate surgery. Trusting my gut and knowing myself was crucial that day.

TIP: Trust your own feelings and connection to them. There is no one who knows better than you about what your needs are.

Afterwards, I slept and slept and slept for days, trying to find some state of oblivion to make it not real. Being awake was agony. When I woke, I would cry until I was thirsty.

And then it happened again. After number two, I went to see the reproductive endocrinologist whom I had seen five years prior when we struggled to get pregnant with our first child, my oldest son. I was told at that time that I had the reproductive system of an eight-year-old girl. It took three pretty easy (relatively speaking) rounds of injections, a few rounds of acupuncture, and timed intercourse (IUI). My beautiful dream came true when he was born. We were told that we would need to follow the same procedure when I wanted to get pregnant again, but in a hilarious (and terrifying) twist of fate, I got pregnant the precise moment I stopped nursing my son. I knew that I wanted another baby but was gun shy given how taxing the few short months it took to get pregnant the first time were.

TIP: Seek advice from a professional, including a second opinion. this was crucial in feeling confident enough to move forward.

I had my daughter 15.5 months later at 34 weeks. Her birth was a horrifying and nothing-but-miraculous grade two placental abruption, but she, by the grace of a higher power, lived and thrived. We were told if we had waited another ten minutes to get to the hospital, we would have been burying her instead of babying her. This event - my daughter surviving - provided me with both conflicting faith and absolute horror when thinking about the future. Both babies were born by emergency c-sections. They had taken my daughter out literally just minutes after I began hemorrhaging and before she'd have drowned in my blood. Minutes. Maybe just one or two. I often wondered if I was pushing my luck and being selfish in thinking that I could have a third and maybe even a fourth baby, knowing what it took to have these two perfect babies. I supposed I just was not cut out to carry or deliver. But I also trusted the process and my gut feeling (hope?) that I was meant

to be a mother to more than two. I did my research to learn about subsequent risks.

TIP: I strongly suggest getting bloodwork and testing done before to be sure that there isn't anything preventable or treatable being overlooked.

Afterwards, the bloodwork showed no bleeding or clotting disorder, nothing to diagnose-- until the specialist told me it simply was not in the cards. He said that two losses following two healthy pregnancies was indicative that something was wrong. Typically, he said, in an attempt to not communicate complete hopelessness (but communicating complete hopelessness) two miscarriages in succession was not a great sign.

"Low ovarian reserve" he said.

"Your eggs are aging faster than you."

However, he added, "...this is not an exact science. I am deducing." Then, there was a third loss. And a fourth. Each time, my body held onto the pregnancy, requiring another surgery to nightmarishly remove the dream from within. I stopped believing or even being part of the process. I did lots of tests. A decade ago, my parts were like an eight-year-old's (so young and pristine!); now, they were now functioning similarly, to those of a 48-year-old. My ovaries were aging in fucking dog years.

Woof.

Each loss- one after another after another after another after another- was such a slap in the face because that beautiful ticking metronome on the screen had been there; every-single-time. Every time, the surgery to extract the remaining hope that had settled so securely in me that it refused to budge was taking something from me, from my whole person. I had an incredible support system each time; some who knew this pain, some who would never; but all who wanted me to find my way through. I was more and more hopeless, much less connected, wondering (and making the doctors wonder), if my ovaries were filled with rotting eggs, then why was I able to get pregnant so easily? A cruel trick of nature? Then I unraveled. My marriage began to unravel. I had to actively and consciously say goodbye to the idea that I would ever be a mother to anyone else. I accepted this with a lot of sadness but also exponentially more love and gratitude than ever. Appreciation for the children I had and fury over the ones I didn't were not mutually exclusive. My son and daughter were enough.

TIP: Finding the support of friends---or strangers-- who have experienced similar losses as this will be priceless and affirming. I felt it impossible to explain to anyone who had not felt this pain.

I got divorced -- there was too much pain and distraction on my part to be interested in repairing my marriage. Even though I was very much supported in that marriage, it could never have been enough. My body was broken, wracked and so was I.

I fell in love with my now-husband. We enjoyed our alone time. I had kissed the dream of a third baby goodbye, sold all my baby clothes, sweet with milk and that sweet baby smell, and got breast implants to repair my sucked-the-life-out-of-me-boobs as even further affirmation that I knew this ship had sailed--radical acceptance. I convinced myself that life and God had my shit all worked out and that I should trust it. I had also begun believing in a God that I wasn't sure existed before- I had to; I had to trust that someone bigger was in charge of this all.

TIP: I have always been a spiritual person, but I really worked on thinking about a higher being as the One in control and fought to trust the process and yield to Whatever or Whoever was deciding my fate.

Despite my real efforts to believe it was "for the best". I never totally did. I needed more time to grieve--maybe the rest of my life. I cried every time I was asked about my first loss; and I still do. It knocked me on my ass harder than I could have ever expected. It took me out. It was the first time I actually understood that one could die of a broken heart. I had no idea that the loss of someone I had never known could feel so tragic and take a piece of me like it did. But I had known him. I had.

Whatever I did, my moments were imbued so wholly by these losses that I could focus on nothing else. I was subjugated by these losses; constantly fighting the battle to be grateful for what I have but so, so pissed at what I had lost. Resigning to Mother Nature felt comfortable after some time, and I yielded and accepted all the cliches my friends convinced me to believe. It was better this way. Everything happens for a reason. God has a bigger plan. It was not meant to be.

But perhaps it was meant to be. I had almost forgotten this big dream of mine when I was dating Eric and falling so hard in love that I could not imagine needing anything else. But love is funny. In my daydreamy love state, I was also sad that if Eric and I were to really live this life together, we would not have the opportunity to create a baby of our own; something I believe to be the most intense sharing experience in the world for a couple. We flirted with the subject- but mostly skirted around it, both knowing that it was going to take a miracle and a shitload of money and needles if we really wanted to invest in having a baby.

But the miracle happened without the money or the needles. Without praying and no longer asking the world for it. With each pregnancy, I had known right away that I was pregnant, and this time was no different. For the first time, I didn't want to know or to feel. I had already bid adieu to this pregnancy stuff and had donated my dreft-scented memories to someone else who would create their happy new ones.

I was 39, and my two kids were 8 and 9.5. It seemed impossible but the test was positive, as I knew it would be. I called Eric to the bathroom, and he held me while I fell apart and cried and cried, reliving all of my pain and fear while he re-lived his own feelings of hope and excitement experienced with his own son.

"Don't get too excited; I am going to miscarry," I said.

He never, ever, ever believed that I would...ever. He is stubborn as a donkey (which kills me most of the time), but in this case, it was so affirming and hopeful that I affixed and secured myself to his thinking and went begrudgingly along with it. Then I started bleeding at 10 weeks, but Eric was certain it was a fluke. It was. He knew I would be okay even when I had to go in every month and then every week and then every few days because I was considered high risk (due to my previous placental abruption and also that I was a "geriatric" mother-to-be; kick me when I'm down, why don't you?!). He (frighteningly, but I think joyfully) stabbed me in my growing right glute every Thursday night with a juice-box-straw-sized-needle filled with some hurt-like-hell-serum as thick as corn syrup for a purpose I don't even know. At 26 weeks, we spent a night in the hospital with irregular contractions.

"Go rest. You are stressed and dehydrated."

NO SHIT. I had been stressed for 9.5 years, but this was a new level of heightened fear and anxiety-- even for me. No matter what I was doing-any day, any time - my brain was chanting,

"you're pregnant, you're pregnant, you're pregnant, you're pregnant."

Eleven weeks later, at a day shy of 37 weeks, remarkably (and ironically) very relaxed at my weekly non-stress test, having just come from the gym, the nurses came running into my room doing their best impersonations of calm nurses. But I saw the urgency in their eyes.

"Honey, the doc doesn't love the way this heart rate is dropping regularly; we need to get this guy out. You should tell your hubby to get here in ten minutes, or he is going to miss it."

Well, SHIT, this sounds pretty much like my biggest fear. I only remember

seeing Eric next to me from my paralyzed horizontal position; he was sitting at my head, patiently wiping my endlessly pouring fountain of tears away for two hours. All the thoughts went through my head. This baby is going to die. I am going to die. I am so selfish for doing this. I am going to die and leave my daughter and son (and maybe this baby boy IF he makes it out alive) without a mom. What the hell are they going to do without me? My husband is going to be a 40-year-old widower. I can't do this. I am too old. The world had distinctly told me "No" so many times. Why did I need to try and make it a "yes"?

I am not sure if I am proud or ashamed of the moment that I remember choking back tears and reminding my doctor, without mincing words, to "tie those mother-effing tubes and quadruple knot them." If I lived, I would never, ever do this again.

Then there was a sound I will always remember-- that baby bird, the teeniest five pounder with a voice just trying to get out; a baby squawk. The most amazingly beautiful and surreal sound in the whole world. I fell apart. We both did. (Maybe Eric had been frightened after all.) Our boy was here. We did it.

Just yesterday, I looked at my husband as our baby, Jax, the glue that brings our family together with the strongest bond, was running around like a maniac, and I said, "Can you believe we had a baby?!?!"

"Um, yes, he is a toddler now, and he is nude and peeing while twerking," my husband replied, as we watched all four kids in total wonder. There is not a day that goes by where I don't feel grateful for who this process made me or us or our family. Jax will never make the pain of my losses go away, but it is, without a doubt, a surprising and insanely lucky gift. The pain from these losses always had me wondering which is worse; the shock of what happened or the pain over what never did. But it did happen.

> *TIP: It took a long time for me to be comfortable with feeling both gratitude and loss. I never wanted to feel ungrateful for what I had and the new baby I was given, but I have given my permission to both grieve and celebrate.*

He is the period at the end of the sentence--no pun intended. There are no words that make my heart soar more or more sore. He made me more grateful than I imagined I could ever be for my life and the lives of everyone else in my house. He made my biggest dream become real after I had already decided the rest could only be a nightmare.

With each child, there has been a story; my first required fertility treatment, my second required a total miracle and a crazy-fast emergency c-section, my third, (my stepson) required a few rounds of IVF. My fourth, this sweet baby who changed everything, required hope (and excruciating shots in my bum every Thursday). He required a belief that I never could have imagined I would find. And for that, I am both tickled and intensely appreciative.

Despite how supported and lucky I have been, my struggle left a scar, an anguish and a guilt that I am branded with. It is a trauma that I think of daily.

TIP: The guilt was pervasive. People told me if I hadn't been a runner, or an avid exerciser that it would not have happened. Learning to trust my gut-- and the doctor's words- helped me believe that this was not a ME issue. It was not my fault. Putting the blinders on and trusting only my doctors was important in helping me know that this was not my fault.

I have my beautiful people, and I am endlessly grateful. My story is insidious; I think of these losses daily. The pain, stress, grief, and despair we have experienced is not negated by the gift of a baby. The pain was enduring and isolating and desperate. I thank a higher power every day for being given the chance to finish my story with Eric and to close these chapters. But in my story, there will always be the prologue - an intersection between past and present that my heart will always hold on to. And I will hold on like hell.

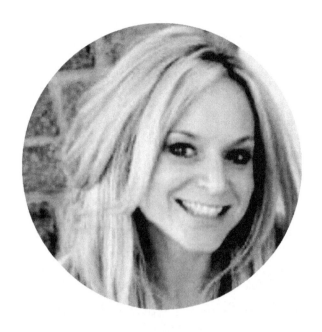

Scan the code for a video message from Jules and a free gift

Jules has been a proud mother since 2008, living at home in Boxborough, Massachusetts, with her husband and their four kids. A graduate and lacrosse player of Connecticut College, 2000, master's degree recipient in 2003 (Simmons Graduate School of Social Work), and chef/caterer by avocation, Jules changed careers in 2012 to become a personal trainer and business owner, being awarded one of Boston's best trainers in 2019. When not enjoying fitness, food, and family, Jules can be found answering the question, "why?" for the thousandth time.

IT'S IN THE GENES

Kendra Becker

had the good fortune of marrying the love of my life. Our courtship and marriage were effortless. We were both in medical school and picked our wedding date because it was halfway between each of our sets of medical boards that were required to complete our studies.

We decided very early that we both wanted children; we wanted to be parents and raise a family together. After a year of marriage, we decided it was time to "try." One ovulation test later, we were pregnant.

Like good medical students, we waited until 12 weeks to make our big announcement at a family Christmas party. We told everyone we were expecting a baby the following June, a month after we finished school. The timing was perfect, and the support and excitement of our families was priceless.

Two weeks later, I had severe cramping, spotting, and pain. I called my provider, the day before Christmas Eve. She said she was sorry; it sounded like I was miscarrying, and there was nothing she could do but send me to the ER. I birthed my 14-week fetus at home, we held him, and then, I proceeded to hemorrhage.

My husband scooped me up and took me to the ER; I was calm but weak. I told the triage nurse, in no uncertain terms, what had happened in a calm, matter of fact, medical way. She asked me why I was so calm, and my response was, "Would I get better care if I was hysterical?"

The nurse took me to "gyn row." I used to work in an ER; I know about "gyn row," where all the gynecologic problems show up, such as STDs, foreign bodies stuck in the wrong place, and bleeding problems. I was evaluated; I had no blood pressure, a heart rate above 150, and I was dizzy.

My poor husband was beside himself; we lost our baby boy, and now, my husband was thinking he might lose his wife too, the day before Christmas.

The ER doctor was as calm as I was. We talked "shop" a little, and he gave me some fluids and sent me on my way. I was anemic, weak, and totally devastated. The worst part was the next days were Christmas festivities, and all the presents our families had for us were for the baby we had lost.

For my own sanity, I needed to know why. Why did I lose a perfectly healthy baby? Why did I lose him at a time in my pregnancy when I was at low risk? Why me? After a long talk with my provider, we decided to send the baby and the placenta for pathology. Just to be certain, we sent it twice. They mailed me a copy of the results. I opened the envelope, and one sentence was written on thick white letterhead, **"no infection, normal chromosomes, XY."** That was all that was left of my baby. Normal. Gone.

Over the next months, I healed my body and learned to live with a tiny hole in my heart that losing my baby left for me. We were still bound and determined to be parents. As physicians, we did everything in our power to obtain a positive outcome. We read the latest research, followed experts, and let everyone give us advice. Quickly and effortlessly, I got pregnant again. It was not planned but very welcomed.

This pregnancy was different. I felt "less pregnant," less connected to the baby, but, like the last time, I saw my baby's heartbeat on ultrasound at 7 weeks. I felt so relieved. I was taking my vitamins, just as the research had instructed me to, stopped drinking coffee, eating fish, sleeping on my back, or whatever the know-it-all researchers told me to do.

During my 14th week of pregnancy, my husband was traveling for business, and I was scheduled for an ultrasound. I had asked for the ultrasound that week because of my previous loss. The OB happily obliged, and as my husband was leaving, he kissed me goodbye, and I happily told him I would send him a picture of the baby from the ultrasound after my visit that day.

I walked into the ultrasound room, prepared to take a picture for my husband. The tech perfunctorily stated, "There is no heartbeat," and, "The baby looked like it stopped growing at about 11 weeks," just like that. I was numb. I got in my car and drove home sobbing.

I called my husband hundreds of times, and he did not answer. Phones were turned off for airline travel in those days. I paged him in the airport and left a message at the gate for him when he arrived. He never got to his conference; he got on the same plane he just got off and returned home to be with me.

The next days left us sad, angry, and questioning. We were required to go for a more complex ultrasound to confirm what we already knew. Nothing is worse than watching a flat line for 30 seconds that is supposed to be your baby's heartbeat. I was done, simply done with heartbreak, done with the parabola of emotions and done with breaking my husband's heart.

I elected for a D&C at that point and was scheduled the next day. "Nothing to eat or drink after midnight," the nurse told me, "Get here at 6 a.m.; you will have your 'procedure' at 7:45." I was checked in, IV started, and then, we were bumped until 2 p.m.

Now, I'm starving, and my husband has not eaten either. We asked several times when it would be our turn, and the staff just kept saying soon. I suggested my husband go get something to eat, so he could at least drive us home coherently. Of course, minutes after he left, they rolled me into the operating room. I'm alone, freezing, and so very upset. This was my first and, to date, only time I have ever had anesthesia. The procedure took minutes, and recovery was swift; the PACU (post anesthesia care unit, where post procedure patients go to recover for a short time after a same day procedure in the hospital) closes at 5:00 sharp, so they got me out of there quickly! We went home and tried to sort out our next steps. We talked about adoption, getting a bunch of dogs, seeing specialists, and all the heartbreak we had endured over the last months; we tried to come up with a plan. All the while, we had started a medical practice together, and we tried to focus on that. Funny thing was, one of my specialties then, and now, is fertility. So, I was lucky enough to have access to the most current research. I have a genetic mutation called MTHFR, which is a gene that codes for an enzyme to help the body break down folic acid (which is synthetic) and turn it into something useful for the body to use in over 1100 metabolic processes, called methyl-folate. Everyone in my family has this gene mutation, my parents, grandparents, and my husband. As a doctor who studies genes and genetics, I thought it prudent to look at my own genes and those of my loved ones. My husband and I did genetic testing while in medical school, and I offered the same testing to my family members who were interested, so I was able to look at everyone's genes. This is how I was able to come to understand my own genetic predisposition. The importance of this gene in pregnancy is the methyl folate helps with cell signaling in the development of a fetus. In my body, the enzyme is impaired and only works at 40% of its capacity. This means I only get 40% of the efficiency of a body that doesn't have this mutation, and my weak point was in fetal development. My body could signal development in my babies only up to a certain point, then it stopped working, and my babies stopped developing. At the time of my miscarriage, the current research showed that giving high amounts of folic acid to women with MTHFR could help. In my first two pregnancies, I dutifully followed the recommendations by the experts. However, while I was gathering information for a case I was reviewing, I received an email from the wholesale manufacturer of my supplement line, the one I created for my patients. My prenatal vitamin was part of this line and was the precise vitamin I'd been taking. I had created the formula myself with the most optimal nutrient levels available according to current research. The email provided the most up-to-date research about MTHFR and folic acid. I was stunned as I read that folic acid could actually HARM a mom and baby if taken in pregnancy if the mom carries an MTHFR mutation. I was taking what the science had shown two years ago to be valid and helpful, and just like that, new research, new findings, and new outcomes! My first feeling was anger. How could they, all of the sudden, find new research!? My thoughts quickly turned to how many women were like me, suffering losses needlessly. In my own case, I thought, "Whoomp, there it is!"

I quickly reformulated my prenatal and removed all folic acid and derivatives from my formulas. Additionally, I started taking more METHYL folate and conceived again. This time, I kept drinking coffee, eating fish, and sleeping in any position I was comfortable.

Tip: Please check my link page for information about my small batch prenatal vitamins. I have chosen only the highest quality ingredients and follow the latest research on dosing amounts.

We waited until 18 weeks to tell anyone we were pregnant; we knew we were having a girl at that point. It was an easy, effortless pregnancy that ended the day before my due date with an uncomplicated homebirth. My husband caught our daughter and was the first person in this world to touch her. He is also listed as the doctor on record on her birth certificate.

MTHFR can affect babies, too. Babies can have poor weight gain, struggle with nursing, be fussy and slow with motor development. I looked for all of these in my baby girl. None were there! She developed beautifully and was and is a healthy thriving young lady. My husband and I briefly discussed having a second child. I did not want to be the mother of just one child, and our daughter was growing so quickly. I missed the baby she once was. He agreed it was time for another and that we probably should start "trying" because we suspected it might take some time to conceive again. It didn't. I strolled into our office one day in January and grabbed a prenatal vitamin off the shelf; he turned to me and said, "Who is that for?"

I said, "It's for me. I need it; I'm pregnant, again."

He responded, "You're pregnant? I didn't even try!!"

This pregnancy was equally easy, and our son was born at home in the water, on his due date, just after midnight. He was a strong, robust 8 ½ pound baby that rolled over at about one hour old. We noticed a dimple on his backside at birth. This was a sign that he could also express the MTHFR gene, so we watched for signs in him as he grew up. He had a tongue tie, which is commonly associated with an MTHFR defect; luckily, my husband is a chiropractor, and he addressed his issue early on and managed it effectively. The only other thing that cropped up for him was some reflux as an infant. Since I was breastfeeding, I modified my diet and removed some items that his tummy wasn't quite ready to digest, so that also quickly resolved. He is now a strapping young man and a talented athlete.

> *TIP: In general, people can live a perfectly healthy life with an MTHFR mutation and never know. Because MTHFR is part of the detox pathway, it may only appear when there is a weakness or imbalance in the body. Common signs and symptoms that bring patients into the office are fatigue or a "feel terrible since..." some incident, illness, or exposure.*

I continued to take a prenatal with methyl folate until my son was weaned. He was our last child, and after nursing was over, I stopped my prenatal and switched to another formulation of methyl folate to ensure that my cells have what they need to function properly.

It is important for me to "mind my genes," even though I believe that our genes do not define us. Our environment (epigenetics) has a far greater influence over our health outcomes.

For us, losing two babies was heartbreaking. I have told my fertility story of my rainbow babies all over the world. If there was one thing, I wish parents would know, it's DO YOUR OWN RESEARCH!! Decide what is best for you. Most doctors are pretty smart people, but you have a PhD in you! There is no "one size fits all" in medicine and certainly not in creating your family. When there are no answers, keep looking!!

To me, there is no greater gift than when a couple comes into my office after being told they can't *ever* have a baby, or they have "unexplained infertility," and then have a healthy baby of their own, simply because we looked at genetics and epigenetics in a different way than another doctor would have.

For our journey, looking deeper into my MTHFR mutation and properly treating it allowed us to create the family of our dreams. Knowing that 60% of the population carries this mutation, it can be a factor in fertility challenges. For us, we are grateful that we discovered this issue and treated it properly. Research is always key. As with everything, there is a study to contradict a study, but choosing to talk to experts and read reliable research helped us find the best path for us.

As sad as it was to lose two babies, I am so grateful to help couples in my practice potentially avoid the heartbreak we endured. Knowing what is in the genes made a world of difference for our family.

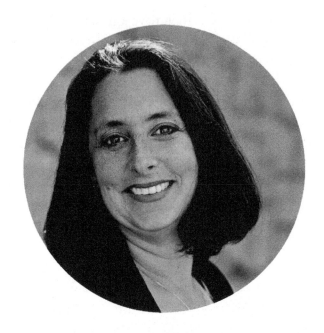

Scan the code for a video message from Kendra and free gift

Dr. Kendra Becker has an integrated doctor of naturopathy (University of Bridgeport) and advanced practice nursing degree (Sacred Heart University) to provide the best possible care to her patients. Dr. Becker understands the importance of integrating conventional and holistic medicine and the importance of combining therapies appropriately.

Prior to becoming a physician, Dr. Becker spent 10 years practicing as an ICU nurse for both adults and children, specializing in cardiac surgery and cardiac anomalies, before studying naturopathic medicine.

Dr. Becker believes in healing through genetics and specializes in treatment of conditions such as asthma, autism, allergies, and eczema, as well as fertility. Dr. Becker integrates both a conventional background with homeopathic, naturopathic, herbal, and dietary treatments.

Dr. Becker is a published author of two books, lectures on various topics throughout the nation, has made various TV appearances to discuss the importance of root cause medicine, and is a member of various organizations.

Dr. Becker is the mother of two healthy children and lives on a farm.

https://linktr.ee/Drkendra

ONE PRECIOUS LIFE

Nancy Powell

My story begins before I ever thought of having children -- in my teens when my cycle was irregular. I didn't know this might be an indication of something wrong with my reproductive system. I was grateful to not have to deal with a period every month, as some months, the cramps were excruciating.

I continued in blissful ignorance until my mid-twenties when I was a blushing bride-to-be and realized I better do something about birth control before getting married. I was already lackadaisical about other daily prescription pills I had to take, so taking a daily pill was not going to be my best choice.

A friend recommended an injection called Depo-Provera. It's a shot taken once every three months that would prevent my cycle and make pregnancy impossible. Having to remember something only every three months sounded like a great idea, so I made an appointment and told the doctor what birth control I chose. I was asked zero questions about my cycle history and received the first shot a month before my wedding.

Three months later, I returned for my second shot, which turned out to be my last. In those few months, something began to wake inside me. I decided I didn't need intervention to put off pregnancy until we were ready to start a family. The idea of overriding my body so completely began to sound drastic. Never before had I been in tune with my body, but something about these injections seemed unwise.

TIP: Despite choices you have made in the past, it is NEVER too late to make changes!

Whatever the catalyst was that caused me to discontinue the shots, I am thankful. The shot didn't simply skip my menstrual cycle for three months. My cycle stopped for over two years.

On our second anniversary, my husband, Mark, and I went to celebrate and have some conversation about marriage so far. We'd already had ups and downs, adventures together, were happy in our steady jobs, and realized that we were ready to start a family! I can still picture sitting there, knowing that it was one of our most special days because we made the decision to start a family.

I knew there was an obstacle to overcome on our way to pregnancy and parenthood; I still had no menstrual cycle and hadn't since before our wedding, even though the last shot I took was two months after getting married. I hadn't been concerned before because I was not trying to conceive. Now what? I'd grown wary of doctors, knew no one who had been through a similar situation, and didn't have social media to turn to for advice. I felt alone.

Eventually, I did turn to the internet, although my searches were fruitless at first. I had to learn from old-fashioned message boards and dig for information. Finally, I came across a few people who had taken the same shot and had the same result. One person shared how she had gotten her cycle back after going on a raw diet.

I was skeptical and wondered if I would ever be able to eat that way, coming from a standard American diet. I gave no real thought to what I ate. Could I now shift to intentional decisions about everything I put in my mouth? My maternal instinct overrode all my hesitation. I had a starting point. What was a raw diet and how could I start?

I started the raw diet, imperfectly and temporarily, and still saw results. This was my first big experience that doing *something* for your health produces good results. Nowadays, there are lots of resources to make amazing raw meals. But for me, eating raw then meant avocados, bananas, nuts, and slightly warmed tomato soup. I cannot claim that what worked for me works for everyone, but those enzymes or nutrients that I got from raw food were a huge piece to my puzzle. Three weeks after my foray into eating raw (with a few cheats), I got my period for the first time in over two years!

TIP: Do not let perfection stop you. Some improvement is better than no improvement.

The next several months included prayer, timed intimacy, and a new hobby of buying pregnancy tests whenever there was the smallest chance it could be positive. It was also filled with many pregnancy announcements, baby showers, and newborn arrivals in our group of friends. We rejoiced for each precious life, and I am thankful to God for a lack of bitterness or envy toward anyone receiving the blessing for which we longed. While my heart ached to start a family, getting to share in the happiness of friends was a grace.

I kept celebrating others, counting days on the calendar, buying more tests, and then, one day, it was positive. I was pregnant!

Seeing that second line on the pregnancy test after taking dozens of negative ones was surreal. I thanked God, shouted for Mark, and quickly took another test "to make sure." It was definitely positive, and life started changing.

The biggest change that happened was getting off my daily prescription to support my neuromuscular condition. Not having this medication was a huge unknown. Even though I'm an optimist, I was a little scared.

When I was six, I woke up one morning and could not sit up. At the hospital, I was diagnosed with a periodic paralysis. Without proper care, my body could get weak in varying degrees up to and including full paralysis. Triggers include *not taking the medicine*, diet, exercise, and stress.

The prescription I decided not to take was a class C medicine, and I had to dig deep for information why. After researching, I decided to forgo the prescription during the first trimester when certain fetal developments occur.

Not taking the medication put tremendous strain on my muscles, and I experienced a lot of weakness. I was working for an investment firm in downtown Washington, DC, and riding the Metro to work. While I loved my work and my colleagues, I still found the work stressful because of the nature of the business.

A few weeks into my pregnancy, I went to use the bathroom and could not stand up. My legs had gotten too weak to push me back up. I eventually made the decision to fall onto the ground and crawl over to a chair, where I might be able to pull myself back up.

I was in mid-crawl when our office manager, noticing my long absence and being concerned about my condition, walked in and found me on the floor. She tried to help me but had to get another lady from the office, and all three of us worked to raise me to my feet. It was an utterly humbling moment to be found on a bathroom floor and unable to stand. This experience helped forge my inner strength and gratitude for my co-workers with whom I am still in touch eighteen years later.

My husband had to be strong enough for both of us. He left work that day to take me home, where I could supplement with potassium and rest until my body started working again.

The nature of my muscle disease qualified me as a high-risk pregnancy. That meant early and frequent ultrasounds. I remember the spring colors I was wearing, the purse I was carrying, and the joy I was feeling that April day when I went in for our nine-week appointment.

I also remember the extremely long time that the tech, and then our perinatologist, moved the machine over my body in silence. It seemed to last forever. The kind doctor looked so serious. Mark looked devastated. I was in denial and wanted the ultrasound to be over, and at the same time, I didn't because I was afraid of what the ending would be. Unfortunately, I will also always remember when the doctor finally looked up with sad eyes and softly spoke, "Your baby has passed."

I felt instant disbelief. It did not seem real. We had already fought our battle just to get pregnant. The research, the diet, the weakness -- I had experienced "my share" of hardships, and now, the loss of our baby seemed too much to bear.

I don't remember much of the month that followed. Getting through it took my husband and I leaning on each other, our faith in a loving God, friends who gave us food, and, for me, a month of antidepressant pills. After a couple days off work, I had to function in normal life and go back to the office. I am grateful that my doctor knew how hard this would be and suggested a prescription. I took them for a month. At the end of the month is when I noticed the first small hope.

We lived in a small 1936 Cape Cod, and our bedroom had a tiny bathroom. It took two steps to get from the bed to the toilet. In that glamorous location one morning, a month after my miscarriage, I realized my first thought upon waking was not of the day we lost our baby. Every morning until then, it had been my first thought upon waking—even before I could sit up. That day, I realized I had made it from the bed to the bathroom before remembering my overwhelming grief. I knew it was my first small step of healing.

After I turned that corner, the next nine months were filled with the ups and downs of life. We were still sad, but there were happy moments, too. I was busy at work, in church, and with friends. Eventually, we started trying again, now with even more emotional baggage added to the already hard burdens of time dragging on and timed intimacy. Those are not ideal romantic ingredients for marriage, but we knew it would all be worth it if we could grow our family with a child.

The combination of a miscarriage, emotional stress, and heightened responsibility I carried working in the investment firm began to undo the strides I had made in caring for my body. I was trying to put as much joy and convenience as I could into my busy days and had quit paying attention to my diet. My menstrual cycle barely came back after my miscarriage, was irregular, then stopped. I talked with my husband, and we realized we needed to make some drastic lifestyle changes.

Up to this point, the only medical intervention we tried was Clomid to see if that would induce ovulation and kickstart my cycle. It had not been successful, and we decided not to try any more medical interventions. Remembering that it was a *lifestyle change* that had brought my period back before, we focused there.

I paid better attention to my diet, but we didn't stop at just food. Mark had been reading more about chemicals in tap water, so he arranged to have filtered water delivered. I think that was the Holy Spirit nudging my husband to check our water situation. I am convinced that having access to clean water is a necessity for health.

Finally, one of the most dramatic lifestyles changes we made was the decision for me to resign. Staying home was going to lower the stress I was feeling, and we were hopeful that this would help me get pregnant again. Also, knowing that when I became pregnant, I would again give up my prescription supporting my muscle strength, we did not want to put my body through the daily commute. It was not ideal to be working that job while my body's strength would be compromised during the first trimester.

This was not an easy decision for us as it was not only a good and well-paying job, but I also truly cared for my boss and co-workers. Downsizing to one income was a sacrifice, but we had faith that all would work out for our family. Although it was a significant adjustment, it did not take long to reap the payoff. Six weeks after beginning my slower paced, at-home life, my period returned. Hope sprouted.

Six months after leaving full-time employment, I had a feeling that it was my time. Obsessed with tracking days, I convinced Mark that the time was now. Intimacy-on-demand is not an ideal invitation, but I communicated that this was definitely the right time, and it happened. IT HAPPENED. Two weeks later, we rejoiced at the positive test! Almost one and a half years after receiving the worst news of our lives, we now had the best!

A few weeks pregnant, I was anxious about my first ultrasound. As it started, I could tell that the doctor was concerned, although he quickly let us know the baby was okay and had a good heartbeat. We praised God! Then, the doctor shared that the ultrasound revealed a large tumor growing over my organs. I needed surgery to have it removed as soon as I was out of my first trimester. Until then, all I could do was wait and pray.

I experienced both nausea and muscle weakness in those following weeks, but nothing could take away my joy. I was not too worried about the surgery, although I knew it was serious. As risky as the surgery might be, it seemed to be a much safer option to remove the tumor in a planned surgery rather than taking the chance that it ruptured, requiring emergency procedures that risked both our lives.

The day came, and many people were praying for us. A friend of mine had come to sit with my husband at the hospital during the surgery. We were all in the room together when the doctor came back to let us know that the surgery went well and tell us about the tumor. While the surgery was necessary, it had been a dangerous undertaking. She assured us the baby looked perfectly fine. Whew! We were one huge step closer.

However, I was not out of the woods. Having gone through the physical stress of surgery, my body was getting weaker and weaker. I was given potassium by IV, and it was constantly being increased. Baffling all medical personnel, my body kept slipping into near total paralysis. Eventually, the only thing I could move below my head was my thumbs. My blood draw revealed my potassium was 1.4, which alarmed everyone. I was rushed into a telemetry unit to track my heart—it was just about my only muscle still working.

Having made it through a risky surgery, now my baby had to make it through a paralyzed mom whose heart was trying to keep beating. In desperation, a doctor asked me what I do to help myself when I get very weak. I told her I take liquid potassium by mouth with juice, and she told me to do that!

Thankfully, shortly after taking oral potassium, the slide into paralysis stopped and strength began to return. Baby and I had made it!

Months later, after an eventful pregnancy, most of the delivery experience was surprisingly relaxed. Everything was peaceful until, suddenly, it wasn't. An alarm sounded, and many medical personnel rushed into our room at once. The doctor said to me, "We are getting her out now!" On my next contraction, in addition to my pushing, the doctor used a vacuum extractor. It somehow seems fitting that our journey ended with a little extra flair. Thankfully, baby was perfectly healthy, despite her dramatic entrance.

Going through that sort of a fight to start our family changed us. We do not take for granted having a child. We don't wish away hard seasons or let time go by without being intentional. Our family has chosen certain ways of living differently because our family is a gift.

Living differently meant we realized there were many places we wanted to travel with our daughter. There were more places on the list than there were summers left in her childhood, so we quit our jobs, bought an RV, and traveled the country for a year, going to national parks, museums, Broadway, and beaches, and visiting with friends and family from coast to coast. Not all years were that exciting, but we still say "yes" to adventures and make sure the memory bank fills up with experiences.

Another way we choose to live differently than others is by being picky about what we use in our home. Choices in food, water, and lifestyle were an amazing start that led us to our daughter. However, we had not made the shift to making sure all household products were non-toxic. We will never fully know what role that played, but several years later, we experienced a second miscarriage.

That pregnancy happened after I gave up trying to have another child. I was finally at peace with the idea that our family was complete and was then surprised to find out I was pregnant again.

Sadly, similar to the first miscarriage, initial tests and doctor visits looked promising, only to learn weeks later that our baby had passed. We were just as sad going through it again. After that experience, I wanted to learn more about making sure that what we use on or in our bodies would be free of harmful ingredients. Toxins add up and make a difference to overall health.

TIP: Check the ingredients in all your personal care products and household cleaners. Many of them are very harmful to human bodies. Research and choose carefully!

My journey through infertility and, ultimately, to my miracle child holds a lot of grief and tears but also joy and gratitude. Although many of the days held traumatic moments, I can still say that, overall, I'm thankful for what I learned and received along the way. Not only did I receive my miracle baby, now a teenager, but I also gained perspective that nothing can be taken for granted, no opportunity should be wasted, and every day is the best day to live intentionally.

My encouragement is to embrace your one precious life. Keep working for what you want, but do not wait to enjoy life or celebrate until you get married, have a perfect marriage, are pregnant, have the perfect size family, get a boy, get a girl, get a job, can retire, or anything else. Today, this day, is your life. The pain, the joy, and the ordinary make up your days. Learn to love all of them for what they offer. I'm cheering for you.

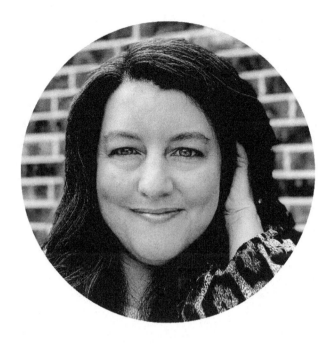

Scan the code for a video message from Nancy and a free gift

Nancy is a fun-loving, action-oriented life coach, focused on helping families create lives filled with fun and freedom. Her favorite days are spent on adventures or making special memories with her family and friends. Reading, traveling and making reels are among her favorite hobbies. Nancy has been to five continents and spent a year traveling the USA with her family in an RV. Her biggest passion is fully living this one precious life and encouraging others to do the same.

https://linktr.ee/nancypowell

A PILGRIMAGE THROUGH INFERTILITY

Jaida Schupp

"Jaida, I recommend you have a hysterectomy." My fertility lifespan was 14 years, start to finish. The average woman has a fertility lifespan of around 30 years. Although my fertility journey was short, I overcame what I was told was impossible. I experienced the heartache and loneliness of going from a child who could not speak for herself and had no idea what was happening to her body to a woman who demanded to be heard. There is something in even the darkest situations that can make a positive in our lives. This is my pilgrimage through infertility.

I got my first menstrual cycle when I was 11 years old; it lasted 7-9 days and was very heavy and very painful.

TIP: Whether you are 11 or 33, period pain is NOT normal. Don't wait to find out what is causing your issues.

I visited my primary doctor, who put me on birth control pills to help with my symptoms and then referred me to an OB-GYN.

The OB-GYN scheduled me for a pelvic ultrasound. The ultrasound came back a little abnormal, but I don't remember being told why.

I had a follow up appointment a few weeks later to have another pelvic ultrasound. The ultrasound confirmed endometriosis, and laparoscopic exploratory surgery was scheduled.

I had tissue removed from the outside of my uterus, my ovaries, and scraped from the inside of my uterus. I had a "string of pearls" around both ovaries. This is where cysts completely outline both ovaries. I was 14 years old.

TIP: No matter the age, you are the advocate for your body. Make sure you fully understand what is being done and why.

Just two years later, I found out I was pregnant. Three weeks later, I noticed some blood. I called the doctor, and they said, if the blood was light and there was no pain, not to worry right away. After six hours, a trip to the emergency room, and an ultrasound, it was confirmed that I was miscarrying.

I laid on the bathroom floor bleeding and crying for days. I would not take anything for the pain; I wanted to feel it all. I could not understand why I was given a baby just for it to be taken away from me right away.

A week later, I had an ultrasound, and it showed that there was still some tissue within my uterus, so a D&C was performed. It was at this appointment that the sentence was spoken which forever changed me as a person. My doctor said that my uterus was tipped at a forward angle, and with the endometriosis, *I would never be able to carry a baby.* This was said to me like it was something that got said every day to everyone, no big deal.

My whole life, I have known I wanted to be a mom. I wanted to have four babies -- two girls and two boys. That dream went up in smoke with one sentence. I was sixteen years old.

Fast forward three years, and my always on time cycle was late. I decided to take a test that evening "just in case." The test said "pregnant." I was 19 years old.

I was getting sick at just the thought of consuming something to eat or drink. I went to an ultrasound to check on the baby and make sure the amniotic fluid was the level it should be because I was so dehydrated. This time, there was a heartbeat. I was relieved but still had some reserved worries because I was only 8 weeks pregnant. The ultrasound tech printed pictures for me. I was also prescribed Zofran for nausea to take once a day.

My belly was measuring closer to 16 weeks than 12 weeks, my HCG levels were measuring higher than "normal," and I was super sick. These are all signs of carrying multiples, but there was only one sac and one baby. The baby was right on track for growth. It was noted that my cervix was a little thin but not too far outside normal, so there was nothing to worry about at this time.

At 19 weeks pregnant, I started having extreme cramping. I was doubling over with tears pouring down my face. I went to the bathroom and checked -- no blood. My husband took me to the emergency room. Less than 30 minutes later, the doctor came into my room. I was having regular contractions every two minutes. I was dilated to 2cm. I was given Meloxicam through IV to stop my labor. Thankfully, this medication worked.

About three weeks later, I went into labor again. We headed to the hospital. I was having contractions every 2-3 minutes, but my water did not break. I again was given Meloxicam through my IV to stop my contractions. Within minutes, my blood pressure and the baby's heart rate dropped. The medication was not stopping the contractions.

After being admitted, I was given tocolytics to stop my labor. I was not dilating, but my cervix was getting thinner. I was given steroid shots to help develop the baby's lungs. On day three of my 5-day hospitalization, I started having regular contractions again. I was given another dose of tocolytics, and it stopped the contractions. On day 5, I was sent home with daily oral medication, another steroid shot, and *strict* bed rest.

At 30 weeks, my doctor wanted to stop the medication to see how I would respond. Within 24 hours of stopping the medication, I was in labor. I was given one shot which stopped my labor. I was sent home to continue daily medication.

Five weeks later, my doctor stopped all medication preventing my labor and took me off bedrest. For two weeks, there were no contractions or any sign of labor. Tired of being pregnant, my husband and I decided to have sex to induce my labor. By 6 p.m., I was able to time my contractions 2-3 minutes apart. I knew from my last appointment that I was still only 2cm dilated, so I stayed home and labored. At 10 p.m., my contractions were just two minutes apart, and there was a lot of pressure. I decided to go to the hospital.

TIP: There is no proof that sex can induce labor, but sex releases hormones that can induce labor if your body is ready.

I was laboring for seven hours since being admitted to the hospital, and there was no change in my cervix. Pitocin was started through my IV.

> *TIP: I would personally go back and try other options before going straight to Pitocin. Continue walking, bouncing on a birthing ball, letting gravity help.*

The doctor did an exam. He believed the baby was in an occiput posterior (OP) position, which was causing my cervix not to dilate. An ultrasound was done to confirm this position. My water was broken, and the baby was manually turned over into a face down position.

> *TIP: Having pain medication or epidural helps relax the muscles when manually turning a baby.*

Two hours after the turn, my cervix was 4.5cm dilated, and the nurse could not feel the baby's head; the manual turn did not work. The doctor decided to try to manually turn one more time. Before the doctor could move his hand from the turn, the baby rolled back into a face up position. I asked for a c-section. He said he would like to see how my labor progressed in the next few hours.

> *TIP: You know your body more than anyone else. Advocate for what you need, not what someone else thinks you should do.*

I had been in labor for 29 hours, and my water had been broken for nine hours. The doctor came in and said I was running a low-grade fever and asked if we could sign the paperwork for a c-section, so if something happened, they could move quickly. He would check on me again in one hour, and if things had not changed, he would take me for a c-section.

Twenty minutes later, my fever was now 105 degrees, and the baby's heart rate was climbing. There were 7-8 nurses in my room, and I was being rushed to an emergency c-section.

Six minutes later, Jordan was born, weighing 8 pounds, 2.5 ounces and measuring 19.5 inches long. She was taken to the NICU for intrauterine infection. Due to her being in-utero when I spiked a high fever, she got an infection from infected membranes, umbilical cord, and/or infected amniotic fluid. She had to spend five days in the NICU to receive antibiotics.

> *TIP: I wish I would have taken more control of my situation with what I felt was right. When I first asked for a c-section, I knew my body was not handling labor correctly. I feel that if I would have stood up for what I felt I needed, my daughter could have avoided time in the NICU. My husband did not know he could have a say in what was happening. We both felt like we had no control over the birth of our daughter, and the plan we had in place was fully ignored in the hospital.*

Six months postpartum, I missed my period. Surprisingly, we were six weeks pregnant.

At 10 weeks, I started having some spotting. It was confirmed via ultrasound that I was having a miscarriage. This was my third miscarriage.

My periods had been progressively becoming heavier over the last two years. The doctor decided to start me on a high dose of birth control to slow the bleeding. Eight weeks later, I missed a period. It was less than one minute before the test said positive. I thought there was no chance of getting pregnant taking birth control.

I had an ultrasound to confirm the pregnancy; I was seven weeks pregnant. I was able to see the heartbeat on ultrasound.

Delivery day! We had to be at the hospital by 5:30 a.m. for a 7:30 a.m. surgery time.

Gavin was born weighing 8 pounds, 8 ounces and measuring 19.5 inches long. In the recovery room, Gavin still had to be monitored closely because he had some accelerated breathing. Within an hour of birth, his breathing was normal, and he was able to eat a little of a bottle.

Three hours later, the nurse came in and told me that she was going to have to start pressing on my stomach. The nurse took my pad and weighed it. A few minutes later, she was pressing on my stomach again, taking the pad and weighing it. Again, just a little while later, she was pressing on my stomach. I thought this was weird; I do not remember my stomach being pushed on this often after giving birth to Jordan. But maybe having a scheduled c-section made something different.

The nurse came over to press on my stomach for a fourth time in an hour, and this was when I finally asked what was going on. She said that I was bleeding more heavily than normal and releasing some bigger clots, so she needed to keep a close eye on it. In less than 30 minutes, there were three other nurses in my room.

My pain medication was wearing off, and my incision was sore. I asked for more pain medication and said, "There is something more going on, isn't there?"

The nurse said, "You are bleeding very heavily, and I have called the doctor. We can talk to her about more pain medication."

Just a minute or so later, the doctor came in. She came into the room and immediately started talking to the nurses, weighed all my pads from pressing on my stomach, went to the computer and looked at a few things, and said, "Jaida I am going to be very blunt with you right now because time is of the essence. You are hemorrhaging and have lost a little more than half your blood volume. I am going to put some medication through your IV to stop the bleeding. I am also going to reach up and swipe the clots from your uterus to slow the bleeding."

It didn't work. She put a balloon in my uterus to put pressure on my uterine wall to slow down the bleeding, but I needed to be ready to go back to the operating room for a hysterectomy, or I was going to bleed to death.

Once in the operating room, the balloon was removed to prepare for surgery. It had slowed down the bleeding, and the doctor suctioned out my uterus and placed the balloon again. She monitored me for a short time and decided my bleeding was under control for the time being, so she was not going to perform a hysterectomy. I did, however, need a blood transfusion due to the amount of blood loss.

Two years later, I missed my period. I took a test first thing in the morning, and it said positive. Just four days after that test, I started bleeding at work. I took myself to the hospital. I had an ultrasound, and it was confirmed I was having my fourth miscarriage.

My periods were heavier than ever before. I was wearing the biggest tampon, overnight pad, and was still bleeding down my legs within an hour of changing my protection. I would wake up in the middle of the night with the bed soaked in blood, and my periods were lasting around 20 days at a time. I told my doctor I could not live like this anymore.

I had a pelvic exam and a sample of my cycle to send for testing to see if there was anything more going on than the endometriosis. I was prescribed high dose birth control to help slow down my bleeding. This had been done before and did not work. My doctor told me these were the steps that had to be taken per my insurance to cover further testing. I agreed; I felt I had no choice.

The results came back, and the blood sample was normal; however, my pelvic swabs came back for possible cancerous cells on my cervix. The doctor explained that he was going to insert a balloon into my uterus and fill it with water; while doing that, there would be an ultrasound being done to see if there were any polyps or abnormalities within the uterus. The issue was he needed this to be done while I was not bleeding, so this made it very difficult to schedule. This appointment took almost three months to happen.

During the ultrasound, the doctor did not see any polyps or anything alarming within my uterus and was able to get the biopsies of my cervix.

My biopsy results came back inconclusive. The birth control was doing nothing for the bleeding, and I was not liking the way it was making me feel. We agreed to stop the birth control and consider different options. I could have another biopsy done to see if those would give clearer results, I could have the cells on my cervix burned off and retested in six months, or I could do nothing and wait six months to see what happened.

Due to my bleeding, he wanted to burn the cells off my cervix, as well as scrape and then burn the lining of my uterus to see if that would stop my heavy bleeding. I agreed to this procedure.

> *TIP: After all the testing and no answers, I should have gone for a second opinion. Another doctor may find something that has been overlooked.*

There was a significant amount of endometriosis tissue within my uterus, around the outside of my uterus, and crushing my ovaries. The doctor was able to remove a lot of the tissue and burn my lining and cervix like originally planned.

Several months passed, and nothing was changing, only getting worse. My cycles were getting longer with each one. I was averaging 30 days of very painful bleeding, with 10-15 days in between. I was sobbing and asking the doctor to take it all; I cannot live like this anymore. The doctor said that because of my young age (25 years old), the insurance would throw a fit. We decided to do another biopsy on my cervix. He asked me to keep records to see how much blood I was losing with each period.

The results came back on my cervix positive for precancerous cells. My doctor was going to submit to the insurance for a hysterectomy. This was going to be a big fight with them, but he felt, at this point, it was my best option. Due to the endometriosis growth, the pain that I was having, the heavy bleeding that we were not able to get under control, and my mental health concerns, he was recommending this surgery.

Two months passed, and I was on day 40 of bleeding, not even able to make it 20 minutes between changing my protection. I went to the doctor and told him I needed this surgery now, or he could check me into the hospital because I was not a safe person for myself.

I showed the doctor my journal of the information as to how much blood I was losing and the pain levels I was having. He agreed that this surgery needed to happen. However, the insurance had denied my claim. He told me it would cost me nothing because he was going to cover this surgery, even if the insurance denied it again.

HYSTERECTOMY DAY

My doctor said, "Your insurance has agreed to pay for this surgery. I got that information two days ago."

Relieved, I was ready for this to be done. My surgery lasted almost four hours. The doctor removed as much of the endometriosis tissue in my abdomen as he could. Due to the nature of this surgery, I had to stay overnight at the hospital to make sure there were no complications. My doctor explained that there was something more going on that went undetected during all the testing.

TIP: I feel that if I would have had a second opinion, this may have been detected sooner and could have been fixed before it became unfixable.

My uterus incision did not close all the way after my c-section with Gavin. This small part was still bleeding and slowly dripping blood into my abdomen and uterus. This could be part of the reason for the heavy bleeding, but the pain I was experiencing was from endometriosis. The tissue had more than doubled from the amount he removed just a year earlier. The tissue was squeezing and crushing my uterus.

I would not have been able to avoid this surgery in the long run. My recovery went very well, and for the first time in many years, I was able to leave my house without worry.

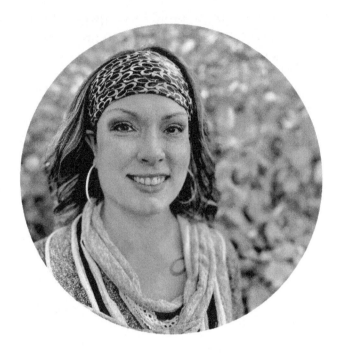

Jaida was born and raised in Iowa. She lives in the Midwest with her husband, two children, and three dogs.

Jaida is currently a vice president of a successful construction company. She is living out a dream for her late father by continuing the construction business he was teaching her before passing. Jaida has also owned and operated a successful daycare business for 10 years. She has begun to write full time and is looking forward to telling her story.

When Jaida is not writing or running a business, she enjoys traveling, baking, and decorating cakes/cupcakes and, if given the chance, seeing a musical at the theater.

MUSTARD SEED IT

Jennifer Tunny

S ix years? I think?

To be honest, I kind of lost track of how long we struggled with infertility. I know a lot of people could tell you down to the minute how long it's been, but I'm not one of those people. Maybe it's a coping mechanism. Maybe it's a way of protecting my hurting heart. Or maybe it's both. All I know is that it was easier for me to get through that time without focusing on the numbers.

Our story begins in the fall of 2012. After using natural family planning (NFP) for two years to avoid pregnancy, my husband, Jesse, and I decided it was time to start a family. I had been tracking my cycles for years, so I knew exactly when the best time to try was. I had no doubt we would be pregnant right away. Oh, how naïve I was.

The day after we tried for the first time, I thought I felt some cramping. "This is it! I'm pregnant!" I thought. I calculated a due date. I dreamed of first birthday parties. I imagined being pregnant in the summer. My mind went crazy.

Finally, it was a few days before my period was due. I hadn't seen the temperature shift that usually happens when pregnancy is achieved, but I took a pregnancy test anyway. Negative. My heart sank, but I remained hopeful. I told myself it was still early.

Then, my period came. My heart sank again. I told myself it was no big deal. We would try again. My doctor told me that it usually takes a few months to conceive, so I convinced myself I was crazy to think it would have happened on the first try for us.

The second month came. I had years' worth of data on my cycle. I knew the differences between sticky, creamy, egg white, and watery mucous. I had been taking my basal body temperature (BBT) at 6:00 a.m. for years. I *knew* the best days to try. Surely, it would happen this time. Nope. No temperature shift. Another negative test. Another period.

And the cycle continued ... for months. Every time, a negative test. And every time, a broken heart.

About eight months into our journey, I had my yearly check-up with my gynecologist. He asked how things were going. I told him we hadn't seen a positive test yet. He suggested a hysterosalpingography (HSG) to ensure that my fallopian tubes were open and there were no blockages.

I went for the HSG the following month. The lady performing the scan told me she saw women get pregnant just from having the scan, even if there weren't any blockages. A few days later, I received the news that my tubes were open and there were no blockages. I clung to the words of that sweet lady and hoped that maybe the procedure alone would be enough to allow us to conceive.

It wasn't.

Month after month went by. I still tracked. We still tried. I pleaded for my eyes to see a temperature shift on my charts each morning. I didn't. I bought the OPKs. I tried the ovulation microscope. Still, not a single positive pregnancy test, so I finally just stopped taking them. I could handle the tracking. I could handle not seeing the temperature shift. I could not handle seeing the negative test result every month, so I stopped. I vowed that I would never take another pregnancy test until I missed my period.

That decision alone made me feel so much lighter. I don't know what it was about those stupid tests, but they were so depressing. I also eventually stopped tracking my BBT, too.

TIP: Do what you need to do to protect your mental health.

It was time for another yearly check-up with my gynecologist. He was aware of my personal beliefs and knew I was not interested in any kind of treatment that did not coincide with them. He was incredibly respectful of my decision but shared that there wasn't much else he could **offer** to help me.

I left that appointment feeling defeated but was determined to find answers.

As part of our marriage prep, my husband and I attended a class on natural family planning. That's where we learned the sympto-thermal method we had been using for years. However, we also learned of something called natural procreative (NaPro) technology during that class. I hadn't looked into it but remembered hearing that it could help with infertility. So off to Google I went.

> *TIP: NaPro technology is designed to work with a woman's body to uncover and treat the underlying cause(s) of an issue. It is a great natural approach.*

I spent the next few months researching NaPro technology. I couldn't find much. I found a website that gave a brief description of what it was, but I was still confused, and I couldn't figure out how to connect with someone to learn more. I felt defeated, and I convinced myself that, eventually, it would just happen.

But it didn't.

Finally, in December 2016, I got serious about connecting with someone. I found a website that listed a few names and emails. I typed out an email, but I was nervous to send it. I was so afraid the answer we were looking for would end with us being told we could never conceive. As long as I didn't have answers, there was still a chance that we could. But if we found out why and nothing could be done? Then, I'd be crushed.

Shortly after I sent the email, I got a reply. My heart jumped! I was so excited to finally move forward ... until I read her email. She was too busy to take on anyone new. My heart sank, and my stubborn self went back to the "we will just figure this out on our own" mentality, and I did nothing for another year. We were three years in, and I was over it. My heart was guarded. People around me were having babies. I fought back tears at baby showers. And the well-meaning comments from family and friends were getting oh-so-hard to take.

> *Tip: It's perfectly okay to take a break from seeking treatment and/or from trying to conceive! This is your journey, not anyone else's.*

About a year after I sent the first email, I decided to try again. I reached out to the same lady. Surely, she'd be able to help me now.

Nope.

Still unable to help me.

She did provide a recommendation of someone else to reach out to; however, I was too proud to do so. The recommendation she provided was over three hours away, and I was set on working with someone local.

> *TIP: You can work with a NaPro technology practitioner remotely! Some services may require an in-person visit, but don't let distance stop you from getting started. https:// fertilitycare.org/find-a-mc is a great place to find a practitioner.*

My ego and I went back to sulking, and I did absolutely nothing (again) for several months. Then, I saw a friend's post on Facebook.

This friend had recently had a baby, and she was sharing about the NaPro doctor who helped her.

I sat there on the couch, phone in hand, staring at her post. I wanted to know more. Where did she go? What did they do? Could I reach out to them? Could they help me? I didn't know her well. Would she think I was weird to be asking her all these questions?

I finally came up with the courage to message her.

"Hi there! I know this is totally random, so feel free to ignore this message if you'd like…"

She didn't ignore me, and with that message, our lives were completely changed. I was so scared to reach out to her. But my friend, Amber, wrote back to me the same night, and she has been a godsend ever since.

She gave me the info to her clinic. She told me her story. And for the first time in a *very* long time ... I had hope. Just connecting with Amber gave me life. It was a breath of fresh air to know someone else who had walked the infertility road, who had experienced the feelings that I had, and who had seen *success*. And it gave me the encouragement I needed to continue on.

It took me a couple of months to gather up the courage, but I eventually made an appointment at the clinic Amber referred me to.

The moment I walked into the office, I felt at home. There was no one pressuring me into procedures I didn't feel comfortable with. I didn't have to question if their recommendations went against my beliefs. Everything was so ... natural.

The first appointments were uneventful and full of questions and orders for blood work and ultrasounds. They did a full thyroid panel and discovered my thyroid levels were not "low" by regular standards, but they were not ideal for conception. I started taking a natural thyroid supplement to elevate them to ideal conception levels. They did genetic testing and discovered a heterozygous MTHFR C677T gene mutation that increased my risk for blood clots and made me unable to process folic acid. I started an aspirin regimen and swapped my prenatal for one with folate. They discovered that my progesterone was low and prescribed bio-identical progesterone. Ultrasounds confirmed I was ovulating properly, and supplements were recommended to help with mucous production and overall health.

> *TIP: Mucous is incredibly important! If your doctor hasn't*
> *asked you about mucous, ask them!*

Finally, I had answers! After feeling like we were getting nowhere for so long, this information gave us so much hope. Our NaPro doctor said there should be no reason we shouldn't conceive before our next appointment. We drove home from that appointment hopeful and excited and even a little scared! After all this time, could this be it? Could we really start a family?

Nope. Not yet.

We went back to our follow-up appointment with no news, and our doctor was just as puzzled as we were. That's when I asked, "What about endometriosis?"

Endometriosis had been on my mind a lot. I have had painful, long, and heavy periods as long as I've been menstruating. I'd struggle to get out of bed the first few days of each cycle because of the pain. I've had to double up with pads and tampons and, even then, sometimes can't go more than an hour without changing them. I've had brown blood at the end of my cycles, and the bloating would make me look several months pregnant (talk about salt in the wound). But in the months leading up to this appointment, I started questioning my symptoms. When I mentioned them, my doctor agreed that it was likely and referred me to a NaPro surgeon.

> *TIP: I always thought my symptoms were normal and*
> *that everyone experienced them while on their period.*
> *Endometriosis affects each person differently. If you*
> *experience any of those symptoms, or any of the others*
> *associated with endometriosis, talk to your doctor.*

I set up a consultation with the surgeon as soon as I could. I shared with him what I was experiencing, and he felt confident that endometriosis could be our issue. He explained the only way to check for endometriosis is to perform exploratory surgery. If endometriosis is found during surgery and is relatively minor, it can often be removed at the same time. If it is major, then a separate surgery would need to be done to remove it. He also explained that he would use excision (not ablation) to remove any endometriosis. That meant any endometriosis he found would be completely removed from my body so that it could not reattach elsewhere. We scheduled the surgery as soon as possible.

I have never been more excited to have a surgery in my life. I wanted the surgeon to find something that would help explain everything. It wasn't that I necessarily wanted to have endometriosis; I just wanted answers.

Four days after my 34th birthday, I had the surgery. The surgeon performed a diagnostic laparoscopy, diagnostic hysteroscopy, and a selective HSG, all at the same time. The selective HSG (different from the standard HSG I'd had years prior) revealed that both of my tubes were open. A sample from my uterus revealed possible infection, so I was placed on antibiotics as a preventative measure. And three different spots of endometriosis were found and removed.

The surgeon said there should be no reason we wouldn't be able to conceive and that it could take a few cycles after surgery. We were excited, but we had heard it before.

Other than some strange swelling in my leg, recovery from surgery went well, and I was back to normal within a week. I restarted limited tracking of my cycles when we met with our NaPro doctor the first time, so we were cautiously excited to see what the next few months brought.

About five weeks after my surgery, I started spotting. My period was due in a few days, and I had no idea what the surgery may have done to my cycle, so I assumed it was starting early.

But the spotting stopped after a few days … and it never started back up.

I *very cautiously* thought to myself, "Could this be it? Could I be pregnant?" I shrugged it off. No way. I was not getting my hopes up again.

A week went by from when my period was supposed to start, and still nothing. I felt a little weird, too. "Could this really, be it?? It had only been one cycle since surgery. There's no way," I thought to myself.

I had stuck to my promise to never buy another pregnancy test until I missed my period, so I didn't have any. I picked one up but was too scared to take it. I wanted to know, but I didn't want to remember that terrible feeling of seeing a negative again. As long as I didn't test, I could imagine I was pregnant.

I finally took the test. It was positive before I could set it down. IT WAS POSITIVE! I couldn't believe it! After all the years of no answers, all the negative tests, all of the questioning, we were pregnant!

As excited as we were to finally be pregnant, it wasn't an easy road for me. My pregnancy was hard physically and even harder mentally. I was scared of something going wrong. I was terrified of losing the baby we had hoped and prayed for so very long.

I started spotting around six weeks, and I almost lost my mind. I knew if I was losing the baby, there was nothing I could do, but the thought consumed me. I Googled for DAYS. I thought about nothing else.

Eventually, the spotting went away, and an ultrasound confirmed all was well, but the fear never did subside. If I bumped the counter, I panicked. If I jumped too high, I worried. If I stressed, I stressed about stressing.

As each month went by, I praised God day in and day out for the little miracle growing inside, but I couldn't completely shake the fear. It was this annoying little voice in my head saying, "Don't get too excited; this could all be taken away."

But our God is bigger than all the fears I had, and at 41 weeks, I birthed the most beautiful baby girl I've ever seen.

Not until the moment that babe was placed on my bare chest did the fear subside. But even then, it was replaced with a new version. Now, as a momma, I still worry about her wellbeing, but perhaps, what I fear the most these days is missing out on a moment. I want to remember them all.

Six years of infertility provided a lot of time to think about how I wanted to do things if – God willing – I was given the chance to be a momma. In those long days of yearning, as my heart ached when I heard folks complain about their kids keeping them up all night or the mess they made, I promised myself I wouldn't complain. I promised myself I would do my best to appreciate every little moment. I wouldn't take one for granted. I would cherish the good days *and* the not-so-good days. I would see the world through her eyes. I would make the memories. I'd overlook the mess. I'd take a slower pace. I'd appreciate sticky hands and messy kisses and interrupted dinner conversations. I would be grateful for bathtub splashes, toys taking over the living room, and sleepless nights spent snuggling the sweetest little soul.

And I do. I'm not perfect, and at times, I still catch myself with my mind too focused on the dirty dishes or laundry that's piled high or the to-do list I haven't looked at in days, but for the most part, I cherish it all.

Going through infertility was hard. And it challenged me in so many ways.

It challenged my patience. I was used to working hard to get most things I wanted in life, but no matter how hard I worked to conceive, I couldn't make it happen.

It made me question what I had done to deserve such "punishment." Why was this so easy for some? Did my husband and I miss our chance by avoiding pregnancy at the beginning of our marriage?

It challenged my faith. God had carried me through the darkest times in my life, and I knew He would carry me through this, too, but what if His plan wasn't my plan? I clung to Matthew 17:20 - "Amen, I say to you, if you have faith the size of a mustard seed, you will say to this mountain, 'Move from here to there,' and it will move. Nothing will be impossible for you."

"Mustard seed it" became my mantra.

Infertility stretched me, broke me down, and built me back up again. But in all of the ways it challenged me, it also strengthened me. Because of the challenge that infertility was, I am more patient, kind, and caring. I know nothing caused us to "deserve" this struggle. And my faith has never been stronger.

Infertility was a dark, lonely road to travel, but as I stand on the other side of it now, I'm so very grateful for the journey that it was, the lessons that it taught me, and the sweet baby girl it led us to.

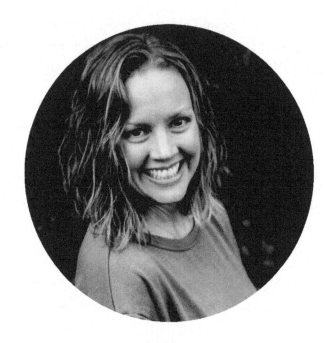

Scan the code for a video message from Jennifer and a free gift

Jennifer Tunny is a small-town homebody passionate about spreading hope through infertility and sharing about the wonder that is NaPro Technology. She graduated from Indiana University with a communications degree and spent 11 years working in corporate America before exiting that world and starting up a small business with her husband, Jesse. These days, you'll find Jennifer working beside her husband in their custom woodworking shop during the day and spending her nights snuggling their sweet baby girl, Gabriella. Jennifer and her family live amongst the cornfields of southeastern Indiana on her family's 100-year-old homestead.

ACKNOWLEDGMENT

This book could not have happened without my incredible husband Roy "running interference" on the home front while I worked on the book. Thank you for always being my biggest cheerleader and believing in me. I love you so much for saying yes, every day to our crazy life. To Kingston, Bronson, Preston and Holden you inspire me every day to be a better human and I'm so grateful to be your momma.

Thank you to my publishing mentor Meggan Larson for showing me the way and to my business coach Martha Krejci for "getting off the couch" all those years ago so my dreams, these authors' dreams and our readers dreams can come true. You're a remarkable human being and I'm grateful to know you.

A special thank you to all the authors for believing in the project and opening your hearts and deepest wounds to the world in hopes of sparing another woman the same.

Thank you, dear reader, and please know we are ALL praying for you, and voting your victory. Praying the breath of God, breathed on you.

Made in United States
Orlando, FL
29 April 2022